THE ULTIMATE GUIDE
TRAIL RUNNING AND
ULTRAMARATHONS

EXPERT ADVICE, AND SOME HUMOR, ON TRAINING, COMPETING, GUMMY BEARS, SNOT ROCKETS, AND MORE

BY JASON ROBILLARD

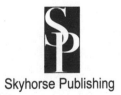

Skyhorse Publishing

Skyhorse Publishing books may be purchased in bulk at special discounts for sales promotion, corporate gifts, fund-raising, or educational purposes. Special editions can also be created to specifications. For details, contact the Special Sales Department, Skyhorse Publishing, 307 West 36th Street, 11th Floor, New York, NY 10018 or info@skyhorsepublishing.com.

Skyhorse® and Skyhorse Publishing® are registered trademarks of Skyhorse Publishing, Inc.®, a Delaware corporation.

Visit our website at www.skyhorsepublishing.com.

10 9 8 7 6 5 4 3 2 1

Library of Congress Cataloging-in-Publication Data is available on file.

Cover design by Liz Driesbach
Cover photo credit Thinkstock

Print ISBN: 978-1-62914-774-1
Ebook ISBN: 978-1-63220-165-2

Printed in the United States of America

CONTENTS

CONTENTS

CONTENTS

CONTENTS

ACKNOWLEDGMENTS

I never would have attempted a project like this if it were not for Shelly's unwavering support and occasional tough love. My life is one awesome adventure after another, and I have her to thank.

Many of the pictures from the book were taken or edited by Stephanie Smedberg. Also, Shelly and I couldn't have done many of our adventures without her assistance.

I have to thank my friends . . . even those that don't really run much. Jesse Scott, Jeremiah Cataldo, Christian and Amy Peterson, Jon Sanregret, Robert Shackleford, Vanessa Rodriguez, Mark Robillard, Phil Stapert, Tim Looney, Jason Saint Amour, Nate Wolfe, Brandon Mulnix, Krista Cavendar, John DeVries, Stuart Peterson, Pete Larson, Mark Cucuzzella, Tony Schaub, Chip Tilden, Pat Sweeney, Bill Katovsky, Kurt Kwiatkowski, Damian Stoy, James Barstad, Mark Lofquist, Gordy Ainsleigh, Emily Snayd, Kevin Mullinax, Ryan Hansard, Dave Repp, Ken Bob Saxton, Rick Robbins, Tucker Goodrich, T. J. Gerken, Michael Helton, Josh Sutcliffe, William Garabrant, Ted MacDonald, Heather Wiatrowski, Shelley Viggiano, Kate Kift, Bob Nicol,

ACKNOWLEDGMENTS

Buzz and Sarah Johnson, Chase Williams, and all the rest of the ultrarunners and friends I've had the pleasure of sharing the trails with over the years. You folks taught me everything I know.

I also have to thank those that helped foster and inspire my creative career, including my parents Gail and Al, Dirk Wierenga, my agent James Fitzgerald, Marianna Dworak of Skyhorse Publishing, Molly Noland, Dr. Cynthia Prosen, Charlie Kohler, Anne Lamott, Don Nohel, Seth Godin, Hugh MacLeod, Chris Guillebeau, Tim Ferriss, Tucker Max, George Carlin, Brian Doyle-Murray, Rodney Dangerfield, Mike Sacks, Chris Kluwe, Melvin Helitzer, Dave Attell, David Ward, Will Ferrell, Mel Brooks, Norm MacDonald, Gerrit Elzinga, Tina Fey, Randy "Macho Man" Savage, Joe Rogan, C. J. Nitkowski, Daniel Tosh, Jack Handey, Steven Wright, and Weird Al Yankovic. I don't know many of you personally, but thank you for shaping me into the person I am today.

INTRODUCTION

Way back in 2005, I caught the trail and ultrarunning bug thanks to a strange mix of pineapple juice, Skittles, and vodka. It started innocently enough. I was teaching high school psychology and coaching football at the time, which had been my "dream" job since my college days. The coaching gig came to an unexpected end (our teams sucked; all of us coaches were basically fired). I was feeling somewhat burned out with football, so my wife, Shelly, introduced me to running.

I had always enjoyed the running I did to condition for football and wrestling, but I had never actually competed before. At first, it was just a component to our weight training routine— it was an activity that helped keep my waistline in check. We decided to add an interesting challenge and entered a local fifteen-kilometer road race. I had no idea that simple, seemingly insignificant gesture would eventually change my life.

Shortly after signing up for the race, we were hanging out with some friends watching the Janet Jackson Super Bowl. Yeah, I don't remember which teams were playing, either. Anyway, after hours of enjoying the aforementioned vodka, pineapple juice, and Skittles cocktails, the conversation drifted to running. Doug Evink, one of our friends, was training for a *twenty-five*-kilometer race later that spring. To us, our fifteen-kilometer race seemed ridiculously long; Doug's race was almost unfathomable. Doug deflected the praise we were heaping on him by changing the subject to marathons. I knew those twenty-something-mile crazy races existed, but thought they were only run by Olympic-caliber running freaks. Doug chuckled at my naivete. He went on to explain that marathons were quite popular and regularly run by otherwise normal folks. In fact, Oprah had run a marathon back in 1994. *Oprah!* If she could do it, I reasoned, it couldn't be *that* unfathomable.

We laughed it off, refilled our drinks, and went back to talking about our training for upcoming races. I more or less dismissed the marathon idea; it just didn't sound appealing. As the night (and drinks) continued, the running discussion died out. We changed the subject to cars, our blossoming careers, and the booming housing market. Soon after the nipple-slip whooping and hollering, Doug turned to me and quietly said, "You know, there are races longer than marathons. They're called ultramarathons. There are fifty-kilometer races, fifty-milers . . . one-hundred-milers even. They're run off road on trails."

That piqued my interest. As a kid, I grew up in a small, rural northern Michigan town. My father was an avid outdoorsman. I spent many days exploring the vast forests near our house and had fallen in love with rolling hills, dense tree cover, the sweet smell of the vegetation, and the sounds of birds chirping and squirrels rustling in the leaves. Prior to Doug's mention-ing of ultras, I had never considered that it was possible to run anywhere besides the concrete and asphalt jungle of our cities and suburbs. I had never considered the idea of running around my childhood stomping ground.

My interest in the idea of trail running was somewhat tempered by the stupid idea of running an incredibly long distance. Honestly, I thought Doug was making up the whole "ultramarathon" thing. At that point, the longest run Shelly and I did was somewhere in the ballpark of five miles. Running ten to twenty times that distance seemed impossible, not only for us but for any human.

When we returned home, the first thing I did was Google "ultramarathon." Sure enough, it was a real thing. I was transfixed. I spent that entire night, despite having to teach the next day, surfing the web and absorbing as much information as I could find. I can't quite explain why, but I knew this was something I needed to do. The sheer stupidity of the endeavor appealed to me. At that point in my life, I had settled into a comfortable routine with moderate, easy-to-accomplish goals. I rationalized the desire to run an ultra as an attempt to fill the void left by the absence of coaching football, and I was quickly consumed by my new "hobby."

Shelly and I ran the fifteen-kilometer race later that spring. They say you're supposed to pace yourself in races—they're right. I committed the cardinal sin of running races: I went out *way* too fast. The race turned out to be the single most painful experience of my life, but I found a weird joy in the experience. I took the lessons learned and began planning for my first ultra. Throwing all common sense aside, I set my goal for a local fifty-miler that very fall. Our daughter was an infant at the time, so I started juggling work, helping Shelly care for the baby, and running.

I'd like to say it was a resounding success, that I performed beautifully and surpassed every goal I had set.

But I didn't.

I spent that summer alternating between long, painful runs and recovering from the injuries from said runs. I would slog around the country roads of Allendale, Michigan, doing my best "zombie limping through mashed carrots" impression. I even resorted to running with Shelly following me in a car, but I found that I got tired. Then I had her drive ahead of me, but found I got exhausted. I went back to solo running.

As the race neared, my longest run was around eighteen miles . . . which was completely inadequate training for a fifty-miler. I made a difficult decision and dropped down to the marathon distance. I managed to finish, but made a slew of stupid mistakes, which included using Mrs. Butterworth's maple syrup as my primary race fuel. Once I came down from the sugar high a week later, I signed up for another dumb race: a road marathon about six weeks later. I managed to finish that race, too, but it forced me to admit something I had never encountered before: the prospect that I might not be able to accomplish the ultra goal. My body simply wouldn't cooperate.

That realization was painful enough to cause panic. And when I panic, I research. Specifically, I wanted to solve the injury riddle. How can I stay healthy enough to properly train for an ultra?

The research led to an unlikely place: barefoot running. As a kid and teenager, I ran barefoot for fun. As it turned out, there were a handful of barefoot runners spread around the country who had used barefoot running to overcome running-related injuries. Feeling like I had nothing to lose, I gave it a try. By sheer luck, I was also beginning a graduate program in educational technology, which introduced me to web design. Since barefoot running was the weirdest thing in my life at the time, I decided to start a *very* rudimentary blog about my experiences as a barefoot ultramarathon runner. At the time, there were exactly two other people that I knew of who shared interest in that niche within a niche, "Barefoot" Ted MacDonald (who would later appear as a main character in Chris McDougall's *Born to Run*) and Matt Mahoney, a dude from Florida.

That initial foray into blogging proved to be a challenge. I averaged six visits per day. The writing was on par with the dialogue from the movie *Showgirls*, the design was as innovative and aesthetic as in the game Donkey Kong, and the comedy was as humorous as in *Dude, Where's My Car*. Unfortunately for you, I've only improved the first two. Despite the amateurish efforts, the blog allowed me to interact with a handful of other like-minded people who were beginning to explore the world of distance running. Those very early online interactions would prove to be a valuable source of new ideas for experimentation, which would become my modus operandi for both barefoot running and ultrarunning

When the Michigan snow melted, I began my ultra training... barefoot. Training went significantly better that year. The barefoot running *seemingly* eliminated my previous injury problems. Later, I would learn there were many other contributing factors, which would radically change how I thought about physical activity in general and running in particular. Finding time was a challenge as Shelly was pregnant with our second child. I had to maximize the unpredictable opportunities to train. The limitations on training and information gleaned from my blogging experiences forced me to embrace the idea of self-experimentation.

The first few months were going well. I had settled into a nice routine and ran when Shelly and our daughter Ava were napping in the afternoon. My plan took a tragic turn in May of that year when my father died unexpectedly. That incredible low was closely followed by the elation of the birth of our son a week later. It was an extremely difficult, busy time.

Running became my solace; it became my therapy. Unfortunately, the babies forced those therapy sessions into the wee hours of the predawn morning. Several days each week after a late-night feeding, I would venture out on a long run at 3 a.m. in the darkness. It was my opportunity to sort out the extreme emotions I was experiencing. For the first time I recognized the emotional value running provided. I'm not an especially spiritual person, but I would occasionally experience some interesting things during my middle-of-the-night runs on deserted trails far from civilization. I would stop along the trail, turn off my flashlight, and sit silently in the darkness. The smells of the leaves, the sounds of the animals, and the feeling of the twigs and dirt would bring me back to my childhood—to a time when my dad and I would spend our weekends searching for animal trails deep in the forest. Feeling his presence in the remote darkness became my coping mechanism; it allowed me to grieve.

Later that fall, I ran the same race I had run the previous year, but bumped up to the fifty. I wasn't quite brave enough to run it barefoot, so I donned a pair of neoprene and rubber aqua socks (those flimsy shoes paranoid people wear at the beach). The race was difficult and I wanted to quit many times. I continued schlepping on more because of the remoteness of the course than my own mental toughness. If I dropped out, I would still have to walk the same distance back to the finish line. Eventually,

I reached the last aid station at around mile forty-seven. I left, made the last major climb, and started hobbling toward the finish. It was then, alone in the forest, that the emotions of losing my father, the birth of our son, and the realization that I was going to accomplish the goal that had eluded me the previous year finally struck me. I was so overcome with emotion I had to stop for a moment to sob uncontrollably. I would later learn that the spontaneous outpouring of raw emotion was a rather common occurrence in ultras. I pulled it together after a few minutes and kept moving.

I managed to finish the race well under the twelve-hour cutoff time. By the time I reached the finish line, I was beaten, bruised, and emotionally drained. The barefoot running helped, but didn't alleviate the pain. My legs felt like Mike Tyson's punching bag. I expected to be elated to finish, especially since I had spent two years working toward this goal. Instead, I was relieved to be able to stop. In true ultramarathon fashion, race directors Steve and Deb Webster provided free beer at the finish line. It was my first exposure to the important association between beer and ultras. I was drinking beer like I was enduring a Cubs game from the bleacher seats at Wrigley. However, I couldn't drink enough to dull the pain in my legs. I vowed never to run this much again.

That vow lasted four days. Once I was able to start walking up and down stairs, I started wondering how I could do better . . . you know, if I were to try again some day. By the end of the week, I had created a training plan for next year's race.

Over the next six years, I'd continue to challenge myself with longer distances and more difficult courses. That crude barefoot blog combined with my fascination with ultras turned out to be a winning combination when McDougall's *Born to Run* was published. Since I was one of the few people who had an active barefoot running presence on the Internet, I became somewhat of an authority on the practice. That led to me writing my first book (the boringly titled *The Barefoot Running Book*).

I'm not a trained writer, but the experience of finishing that first ultra emboldened me to do it. If I could conquer that, I thought, I could conquer almost anything. I took the same approach—I researched various writing methods, practiced (by publishing hundreds of blog posts), used what seemed to resonate with my audience, and discarded the rest. I learned to write what my audience wanted to read as opposed to writing to impress language arts professionals. The first book effort was technically and artistically dreadful, but surprisingly successful. While I would like to chalk it up to genius marketing, the success was probably a function of a large network of generous friends and a weak market for barefoot running books. Eventually that first book led to a second edition, which was later picked up by a traditional publisher. Through hard work, an open mind, and a systematic approach to self-experimentation, I managed to finish an ultramarathon despite limited physical abilities. I used that same approach to become a published author despite having no real training as a professional writer. I can also attribute some of the success to a forgiving audience who laughed at my sophomoric jokes.

That experience eventually led to me teaching running clinics and an opportunity for Shelly and I to leave our teaching careers to travel the United States. We spent almost two years teaching about running form for Merrell, a popular outdoor company. The adventure allowed us to immerse ourselves in the ultrarunning world. We met thousands of runners, ran some amazing races, and explored some of the best trails our country has to offer.

Since I began ultrarunning, I have obsessively researched every nuance of the sport. I would endlessly experiment to get the greatest benefit from my limited training opportunities and mediocre athletic ability. That experimentation has led to many unorthodox solutions to common running problems. I wanted to share these insights with the world, so I wrote a second book titled *Never Wipe Your Ass with a Squirrel*. Due to unforeseen financial issues, the project was rushed. We didn't adequately develop a diverse set of income streams, so when barefoot running slipped in popularity, our running clinic gig ended. I had to publish the incomplete book to pay rent and put food on the table.

The desire to make a more comprehensive guide led me to start *this* project. I received significant feedback about Squirrel Wipe. Many people were disappointed I didn't share more of my own personal experiences in races. Based on that, I included my own ultra journey throughout the book. My goal, though, wasn't to talk about myself—that makes me somewhat uncomfortable. All of us have our own personal struggles we fight to overcome. My experiences with ultras were a struggle, but my heroism pales in comparison to the struggles of an obese person attempting to achieve a healthy weight, the single mother working to feed her children, or a young person diagnosed with multiple sclerosis. Running is just a sport, a hobby we use to occupy our time. I take the sport more seriously than I take myself, but my personal experiences help provide a context for the concepts I discuss throughout.

My goal for this book is to help you learn the basic elements of trail running and ultramarathons by sharing my own experiences. There are no magical shortcuts. You won't be able to simply copy my methods or the methods of your favorite elite ultrarunner and expect instant success. The unique nature of this sport demands that you find *your own answers*. This book will help you find your own answers by teaching you which questions to ask and how to find the answers. This book is about *you* and *your journey* into the world of trail running and ultramarathons. The silliness and corny humor is intentional because I want to remind you that this sport is supposed to be recreation. Take the lessons seriously, but don't forget to have fun. If you're not smiling most of the time, you're doing it wrong. Besides, laughing helps dull the inevitable pain.

Enjoy!

Jason

SECTION 1:
THE BASICS

HOW TO USE THIS BOOK

During my journey into trail running and ultramarathons I encountered a lot of advice. Some was good; some was bad. Much of the advice was contradictory. Occasionally it was counter-intuitive. I found this to be very confusing at first. How could supposed "experts" all develop different methods? Eventually I learned one of the most important lessons a runner can learn: *each one of us has a different path*. It's up to each of us to discover our own path through experimentation.

> *"Life is the great experiment. Each of us is an experiment of one—observer and subject—making choices, living with them, recording the effects."*
>
> —George Sheehan, MD

> *"Adapt what is useful, reject what is useless, and add what is specifically your own."*
>
> —Bruce Lee

These two closely related concepts make up my philosophy of life in general and running in particular. There are *thousands* of variables that can be tweaked in various ways that affect our running. Some people look for the easy answers. They want to be spoon-fed a ready-made training plan, diets found in magazines, or a cross-training routine used by their favorite reality TV "star." They're unwilling to do the work to figure out exactly what works best for them as individuals. That approach usually works well enough in the beginning, but eventually they'll encounter something that falls outside the plan. The results, at least in the realm of trail running and ultramarathons, is rarely pretty. This sport has the potential to cause great injury or even death; you don't want to leave important details in the hands of random strangers.

Mindlessly following prepackaged plans isn't the only problem. Some runners also overreact to scientific research. A correlational study with a small sample size may be published, picked up by the popular media, and unnecessarily hyped within the running community. This happened a few years ago with barefoot running. One particular study was published that suggested a midfoot landing could reduce the ground reaction forces of running. The authors of the research were very careful to avoid overgeneralizing and called for more research before conclusions could be made. Despite this, many runners (and members of the running media) proclaimed the research *proved* barefoot running was best. Even though I'm a proponent of barefoot running, incidents like this cause me to roll my eyes and shake my head. Collectively, our scientific literacy is terrible. No single study is going to provide all of the answers for all of the population. Just because an idea is hyped doesn't mean it's good. The running community is no different than the audience watching Dr. Oz hype wasabi enemas—they declare it to be the next big thing before actually *testing* it. If a single study suggests an idea, by all means test it out. We need to be skeptical and understand the limitations of science.

This book isn't designed to appeal to those looking for a single quick answer. If this describes you, this book is going to be a major disappointment. I won't tell you *how* to run ultras. Instead, I will open a dialogue. I will present you with a wide range of topics and issues ultrarunners face, then give you some insight to the scope of the issues and why they are important. I will toss out some advice based on my personal experience, my research into the science and best practices, and the opinions of other successful ultrarunners. Some of this advice may be useful; some may not. It is up to you to experiment with the ideas, seek out further information if needed, take what works, and discard the rest.

WHY DO PEOPLE RUN TRAILS?

Most runners don't seem to gravitate toward trails until they've already gained some experience as runners. The reasons for exploring trail running are as varied as the individuals who take the plunge into the wilderness. Sometimes runners want to reconnect with nature. Our hurried, frantic lives are filled with noise, clutter, and Starbucks baristas who mispronounce our names. The quiet solitude of nature provides a welcome reprieve from the daily grind. It also adds a degree of authenticity to our closet full of The North Face and L.L.Bean clothing.

Many people seek the solace of trails for health reasons. Trails are usually easier on your body because road running requires monotonous movements repeated time and time again over a hard, unforgiving, unchanging surface. Trail running, with endless variety, softer surfaces, and ever-changing obstacles, gives the body diversity of movement. The health effects are undoubtedly beneficial. Trail running has been an integral part of my plan to live forever. So far, it's worked pretty well.

Occasionally people are drawn to trail running because they've flirted with obstacle courses and mud runs, but Mother Nature provides plenty of naturally occurring obstacles of her own. While these man-made runs offer interesting challenges, getting electrocuted, crawling through mud, and conversing with ab-flexing Crossfit practitioners only provides a finite replay value. You also don't have to pay to use the bathroom on trail runs.

People often turn to trails to seek adventure. Road running is a rather safe, boring sport—the greatest danger usually involves crossing busy intersections or tripping on speed bumps. Trail running, on the other hand, can be quite dangerous depending on location. The possibility of great bodily harm or even death from falling off a cliff, getting lost in an endless maze of crisscrossing trails, or being attacked by a rabid koala bear can be exhilarating.

Others turn to trail running for the camaraderie. This is my favorite element of the sport. By virtue of venturing into dangerous locations, trail runners tend to live by a code. We look out for each other. This results in a sense of fellowship that's difficult to find in other variations of running. It's not uncommon for trail runners to stop and help each other during races, even if it jeopardizes their own races. That selflessness provides a strong foundation for lifelong friendships.

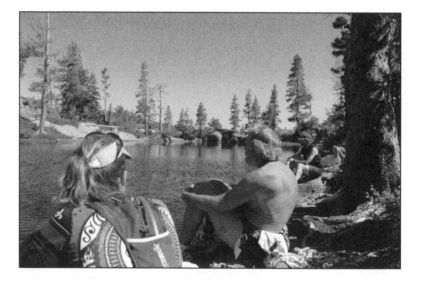

Shelly, Gordy Ainsleigh, Robert Shackleford,
and Vanessa Rodriguez

WHAT IS A TRAIL?

A trail can be defined in a variety of ways. I prefer a simple diagnostic method called the "Christian Peterson test," so named because my friend used to brag about his trail running exploits . . . until he shared some pictures of his "trail." It was a perfectly-manicured path that was smoother than Mr. Clean's head. After teasing him, some friends and I developed the test: *Can you easily push a baby stroller over the trail?* If not, it's safe to call it a "trail."

This definition rules out paved bike paths, crushed limestone trails, and wooden boardwalks. It's not a perfect operational definition, but it serves the purpose. The distinction is necessary because the nontrail trails share more in common with road running. They're a great segue to more advanced trail running. If you regularly run on nontrail surfaces, many of the topics covered in this book will still be helpful.

Technical Trails versus Nontechnical Trails

The term "technical" is used to describe the relative "roughness" or difficulty of a particular trail. Unfortunately, no standard measure exists. When I lived in the Midwest, we called our most difficult trails "technical." Back when I did a lot of barefoot running, I vividly recall teasing friends from other areas of the country. If *I* could run technical trails barefoot, surely they could, too. Then I actually ran other trails around the United States. Needless to say, I was humbled. Our "technical" Midwest trails were like running on an indoor track compared to trails along the Appalachian or Rocky Mountains and the desert Southwest. To help clear up this confusion, I like to use the following definitions:

1. **Nontechnical**: This includes any trail that is free of obstacles or debris. It would be possible to sprint down this trail without worry of tripping. The ultramarathon community sometimes refers to these trails as "runnable."

2. **Moderately technical**: Moderately technical trails have some debris that may require a runner to alter his or her gait. Rocks and roots are the most common. Most of a moderately technical trail is runnable, though occasional walking may be required.

3. **Technical**: Technical trails are covered with considerable debris. Running at full speed may be nearly impossible, but some running is possible. Technical trails may include occasional climbs that require the use of hands.

4. **Extremely technical**: Extremely technical trails are not runnable most of the time. The debris is frequent and dangerous. The trail may require significant climbing with the aid of hands. If you fall on these trails, you're getting some sort of serious laceration or broken bones.

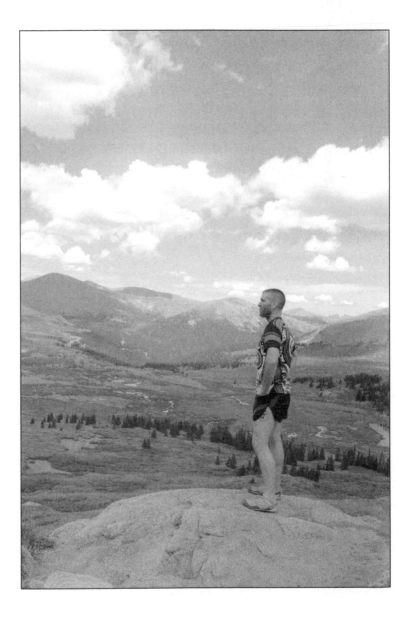

HOW DOES TRAIL RUNNING COMPARE TO OTHER ACTIVITIES?

Trail running shares some characteristics with road running or obstacle course racing, only it's more challenging. It also shares the "getting back to nature" aspect of some activities like hiking, camping, or rock climbing.

Trail running is more dynamic than road running. As mentioned earlier, road running usually involves repeating the same motion again and again for a period of time. You deal with cars, people, and other potentially unsavory aspects of civilization. Trail running adds the element of dynamic movements needed to run up and down hills, through mud and water, and over rocks, roots, and other obstacles.

Trail running is also more vigorous and unpredictable than obstacle course running. Many people transition to obstacle course running because road running becomes too boring and they need a new challenge. Others turn to obstacle course running because they enjoy functional fitness–type activities that require more than just running. These races provide a cardiovascular *and* strength component, which is missing in each individual activity.

Trail running provides more of that experience. Think of trail running as a graduate course in obstacle course running.

Finally, trail running provides the serene nature experience of hiking, camping, and rock climbing without the need for a ton of gear. Trail runners don't carry tents, sporks, and a month's supply of dried chicken kebobs. That lack of gear generally allows for more ground to be covered in a shorter period of time.

TRAIL ETIQUETTE

Lots of road runners make the jump to trail running. This is a great thing! Unfortunately many of these runners carry some bad road running habits over to the trails. I'll cover this topic in greater detail throughout the rest of the book, but here's a quick and dirty (pun intended) guide for new trail runners who are impatient:

- **Don't be afraid of dirt**. I've watched runners in squeaky-white sneakers tiptoe around a tiny mud puddle. I've seen new trail runners on the verge of vomiting when watching a veteran trail runner bomb through knee-deep mud. These are trails. We get dirty. It's a badge of honor; wear it with pride.

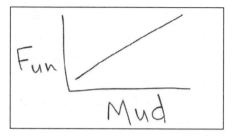

- **Don't litter. Ever.** Don't toss that Gu packet on the ground. Throw your cup in the aid station waste basket. Don't blow your nose and throw the tissue on the trail. *Someone* has to pick up after you, and it's arrogant to expect volunteers to clean up after your mess. It may be acceptable to toss your crap anywhere on the roads, but we live by a different code in the wilderness. Respect our environment.

- **If someone needs help, help them.** If another runner is in obvious pain, lost, crying, or otherwise in distress, stop and help. I've watched the leaders of trail races stop to help others, even if they lose their position as a result. We take care of each other. It's the decent human thing to do.

- **If taking a leak or dropping a deuce, get off the trail.** This one needs no explanation.

- **Be courteous when passing or getting passed.** When passing another runner on a single track (narrow trail), the passing runner should say something along the lines of "passing on the left," then pass *off the trail.* The runner being passed, when hearing this, may step off to the right and allow the faster runner to pass. Only then is it acceptable for the passing runner to remain on the trail.

If a runner approaches another from behind, it's courteous to acknowledge their presence and ask him or her if they'd like to pass. Also, always remember: those going faster always yield to those going slower. Some runners complain of this standard. Don't like it? *Get faster.*

- **Yield to horses.** This is a special case on multi-use trails shared by hikers, runners, mountain bikers, and equestrians. Spooking a jittery horse can be dangerous for the rider and for yourself. Nothing ruins a nice trail run faster than a horse kick to the head. When you see a horse, get off the trail. If you are on a slope, move to the downhill side of the trail. Make eye contact with the rider and announce your presence. Instruct the rider to pass.

- **When racing, thank volunteers.** They're giving their time to *you*. Be grateful. Say thanks. Give them a high-five. Joke around with them. Make them feel appreciated. My greatest pet peeve is to see new trail racers treating volunteers poorly. If you're too arrogant to treat volunteers with respect, please try another sport.

- **Don't expect to be treated like a prima donna.** You're one of many runners running any given race. Making unreasonable demands or expecting people to cater to your crazy-ass needs isn't a divine right. In fact, it makes you look like an ass. And it ruins the day for those of us who want to have a good time. Not surprisingly, expecting to be treated like a princess usually goes hand-inhand with abusing volunteers.

- **Be humble.** No matter what you do, someone has gone longer or done it faster. It's okay to be proud of your accomplishments, but don't talk about them incessantly. Instead of starting a conversation by bragging about your accomplishments, ask others about theirs. You might learn something.

- **Smile.** If you're frowning, grimacing, or expressing any other negative emotion (aside from pain if it's a long race), you're doing it wrong. Cheer up little buckaroo . . . you're surrounded by awesome people and breathtaking nature. Trail running is about camaraderie and mutual support. It's about being a small part of something bigger than yourself. That's what makes it special. You can make your contribution by kicking back, taking it easy, and going with the flow.

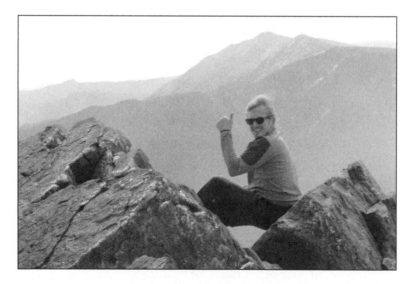

Trail runner Jon Sanregret.

TRAILCRAFT

Trailcraft is the art of navigating a trail using a variety of skills. The goal is to run trails efficiently without wasting a ton of energy, tripping, or falling off a cliff. Road runners have the luxury of largely ignoring their path. The road is predictable. If they zone out or stare off into space, there's little danger. Trail running is different. It requires diligent focus on the path ahead. There are obstacles that present real danger. Rocks, branches, and small woodland creatures all present possible threat. The key to successfully running trails comes down to one idea:

Pay attention to your foot placement!

Ideally, we'd always like to be able to see where we will place our foot with each step. There are three variables that control this: vision, ground feel, and the density of obstacles on the trail.

The ability to see where you're running is important, but not always necessary. With experience and forgiving trails, it's possible to run in complete darkness by relying on the ability to feel the ground with each step. This ability decreases with increased speed and difficulty of terrain. On very technical trails, like the type with sharp rocks, vision is critical. Not only do you have to see where each foot will land but you also have to assure the other foot has a place to land. You have to "see" two steps ahead. If you're wrong about step one and inadvertently step on a sharp rock, you can mitigate the damage by relaxing and taking the pressure off that foot. That requires the other foot to land to maintain balance, which is why you have to assure the second foot has a place to land. If vision is obscured to the point where you cannot "see" that second step, running becomes almost impossible. This may be due to darkness, snow covering hard ice, leaves covering rocks, etc.

Some people have asked why I use a handheld flashlight when trail running at night versus the more popular hands-free head-lamp. The handheld allows me to discriminate terrain better than a headlamp. With headlamps, the light source is close to my eyes. It's nearly impossible to see shadows and depth, which makes the terrain appear flat (2D). With the light source away from my eyes, the depth of shadows allows me to determine the height and shape of obstacles (3D). Also, the ability to quickly move the light up and down and side to side can eliminate ambiguity.

Some people also ask why I spread my arms when running downhill. The quick answer: balance. The longer answer: maintaining balance if I happen to step on something sharp with that first step. If I'm running fast downhill and step on something sharp, the "relax" reflex kicks in and my other foot immediately searches for a landing spot to maintain balance. Since I'm going fast, I'm outrunning my ability to "see" where the second foot lands. If that foot lands on something sharp, I'm fall-ing. The outstretched arms help me balance, which keeps that fall in the "stumble" category as opposed to the "I'm losing teeth when my head bounces off these rocks" category.

Vision is influenced by sleep deprivation and fatigue. Your tired brain's ability to interpret incoming sensory signals decreases as a function of fatigue and sleep deprivation. These are two factors that make hundred-mile ultramarathons so difficult. When vision is reduced or eliminated completely, the ability to navigate technical terrain decreases. At some point, technical trail running with limited vision becomes almost impossible.

Ground feel is *almost* as important as vision. This is the ability to immediately and correctly identify what is under foot. In many cases, this is an unconscious, reflexive action. The millisecond you step on something, your feet identify it as something that does or doesn't cause pain and whether the surface is flat, cambered, or the footing is otherwise compromised. If the surface isn't even, your body reacts by preventing further downward force. If it is pretty good, your body continues loading the foot as your weight shifts over that leg. Also, if landing on an uneven surface, you will know by both the tactile sensation (part of the foot is touching a surface, part is not) and a proprioceptive sensation (foot is inverting, ankle is flexing, etc). These bodily sensations prevent sprained ankles and allow you to run quickly over uneven surfaces.

"Feel" is always a trade-off of wearing shoes versus being barefoot. The protection provided by shoes allows you a larger margin of error with foot placement. However, any protection you gain is met with a corresponding loss of tactile and proprioceptive sensation, which often affects the running form in trail runners. The thicker the shoe, the less ground feel you get. This is the reason shoe selection becomes a tricky proposition—you have to weigh the costs and benefits of an increase in protection versus a decrease in ground feel. Some of the thickest shoes on the market, like many of the Hoka or Altra models, eliminate most ground feel in favor of superior protection. I found it useful to experiment with a wide variety of shoes and develop the ability to run in several different models. Shoes then become tools that can be selected based on the terrain.

"Feel" is also influenced by sleep deprivation and fatigue for the same reason as vision. If you have adequate vision, you can run without any ground feel at all.

The density of the obstacles is more important than the characteristics of the obstacles themselves. I'll use the example of sharp gravel covering an asphalt road. If the gravel is so dense that you step on many pieces with each step, running is easy. You get a "bed of nails" effect where many pointy surfaces are contacting your foot. The cumulative surface area distributes your weight enough to prevent pain or injury. This is why it's relatively easy to learn to run on asphalt.

Running becomes more difficult when the gravel density is thin enough where you always step on a few pieces but thick enough to make them impossible to avoid. The same concept holds true for overly technical trails. Small, sharp rocks usually aren't a problem. Neither are huge rocks. It's the golf ball- to softball-size sharp rocks that usually cause the problems.

HOW TO FIND TRAILS

Finding new trails to explore is easy if you know where to look. When Shelly and I were traveling around the country, we were always searching for new trails in unfamiliar areas. Here are the resources we used most often:

- **Websites** – There are quite a few websites dedicated to documenting trails. Some are specific to one sport like hiking, mountain biking, or horseback riding. Others are more general and include trails of all types. My two personal favorites are trails.com (requires a subscription) and localhikes.com (free).
- **Municipal resources** – Cities, towns, counties, and even some states maintain pages dedicated to their respective trail systems. These resources are usually maintained by the parks department.
- **Trail running friends and social media** – This one is a no-brainer. Friends will probably know your particular tastes and can recommend trails that suit you. They may know of trails not listed in either of the above resources.
- **Local outdoor-oriented stores** – The employees of local outdoor stores, even "big box" stores like REI, are likely

going to be outdoorsy folks themselves. They'll know the local trails . . . and will sell you a map or two.

- **Drive-bys** – We found a surprising number of trails by keeping our eyes open when driving around. Some trails have no obvious trailhead or markings, especially in the eastern and Midwest states. Sometimes these trails were hidden gems leading to spectacular beauty. Other times they led to an abandoned meth lab.

- **Google Maps** – Google's satellite maps have improved immensely over the last few years. At the time of writing, it's possible to zoom in close enough to see many trails that may otherwise go unnoticed. To find trails, zoom in to a large block of wilderness and look for the squiggly lines.

- **Race schedules** – When all else fails, find local trail races. Most race websites have course maps, directions to the trailhead, elevation charts, etc.

PERMITS, TRAIL FEES, PARKING, RULES, AND TRAIL LOGS

Where I grew up in rural northern Michigan, "trails" were more or less two-track dirt roads intersecting large tracts of wilderness to help combat potential forest fires. There really were no rules or regulations. If you wanted to use the trails for anything, you just found small clearings to park your vehicle and, well, used them.

When I traveled to West Michigan, most of the trails were part of federal, state, or local parks. Almost all had dedicated parking lots that required some sort of parking permit. The parks also had rules regulating things like pets on leashes, whether mountain bikers could use particular trails, and hours of operation. It was my first exposure to regulated trail use.

When Shelly and I started traveling the country, we tried to explore as many trails as possible. We encountered all sorts of regulations, many of which were surprising. For example, some trails required multiple permits to park and/or use the trails. Some parks were strict about staying on the trail itself. Others banned all animals. A few more remote parks required minimal gear in case you got lost. Many rugged trails had a log book at the trailhead. At first I assumed it was sort of like a guest book until a ranger told me they use it to determine where people have been if they are reported as missing.

Finding the rules and regulations is easy with the Internet. Public parks almost always have a web page on their respective government unit's website. If the trails are on private land, the business will usually have a website dedicated to the trails. Almost all trails will have the rules and regulations posted at the trailhead. Get in the habit of reading through them when using trails for the first time.

The most common issue we encountered were parking fees. Most trailheads either required a yearly permit that could be purchased at local businesses or park offices or had a self-serve setup at the parking lot. In the case of the latter, the park would have envelopes with tearable flaps available. We'd fill out the required information, rip off the tab to be placed inside the car on the dashboard, and deposit the envelope with the required money in another box. Because we encountered this so frequently, we started carrying a cigar box of one dollar bills labeled "Emergency Gentleman's Club Fund."

FINDING AND CREATING TRAIL RUNNING GROUPS

Running can be a solitary activity, and it can also be a great opportunity to socialize. When Shelly and I lived in Michigan full-time, our friend Mark Robillard organized a group of friends for a weekly run, which we later affectionately named the "Hobby Joggas." We would meet up at the same time at the same trailhead, run anywhere between three and eight miles, then hit a bar or restaurant afterward. We would also do occasional long runs together (see my "Kal-Haven" story later in the book). That group dramatically improved my running performance because it helped me remain accountable for training runs. The group also gave us an excuse to socialize and share tips and experiences.

Finding groups like this is easy in the Internet Age. A Google search of "[your location] trail running group" will likely produce results. If not, *running.meetup.com* is a great resource. If that fails, check with local running stores. Many will organize their own running groups or know of independent groups in the area.

If you cannot find a group, start your own! It's as easy as gathering a few friends and using word-of-mouth advertising to invite others. The process can be facilitated by creating a webpage, Facebook group, meetup.com group, or by placing an ad on Craigslist. You can also inform local running stores of the group; they will usually have trail running customers who will be interested.

TAKING PICTURES

Trail running offers the opportunity to experience breathtaking natural phenomena. This is one of the major advantages of trail running versus road running. Standing atop a fourteener overlooking the Continental Divide is a hell of a lot more awe-inspiring than a bunch of cookie-cutter McMansions, the freeway underpass, and a Kroger parking lot.

Recording these memories is great, but there is a danger in spending too much time documenting and not enough time experiencing. That amazing view from the summit is a lot less meaningful if you're snapping 435 pictures.

When Shelly and I first embarked on our RV hobo running adventures, we took a *ton* of pictures on every run. We knew this was likely a once-in-a-lifetime opportunity and we wanted to create lasting memories. After the first few months, we came to the realization that we were spending more time assessing lighting angles and discussing elements of composition instead of simply enjoying the spectacular scenery. To make matters worse, we had fallen into the habit of posting many of the pictures on Facebook. What initially felt like sharing a cool experience with friends morphed into us feeling more like desperate "look at me" attention-seekers who fed off the envy of our friends at sea level.

Our attempts to preserve the memories were preventing us from creating memories worth saving. After a few discussions we decided to stop carrying a camera on every run. We still took a few pictures here and there, but we no longer felt the need to document each and every new experience. It was a decision we do not regret.

SECTION 2:
RUNNING 101

THE ART OF EXPERIMENTATION

If you do a quick search on the Internet, you'll find a tremendous amount of ultramarathon training tips and advice. You'll find dozens of training plans, philosophies, techniques, and research. You'll also find a ton of information refuting each and every one of those training plans, philosophies, techniques, and research.

What does this mean?

There is no one right answer.

You can follow a lot of different plans and still get to the finish line. You can even make up your own plan out of thin air. It does help to have some guidance though, so how do you choose? I gave some common options earlier. Many are tempted to just do what their favorite elite runner does. This will probably work, but that elite, like every other runner, is a different individual. His or her plan probably isn't the best fit for you.

This book covers a large number of ideas, from broad training plans to the tiny details of ultrarunning. I would highly recommend developing your own process of experimentation to decide how to deal with each issue. Test out a wide variety of ideas. Keep those that work. Get rid of those that do not.

By using this process, you will continually improve using the methods that work best for you.

In essence, think of your ultramarathon training as one huge experiment, and you're the subject.

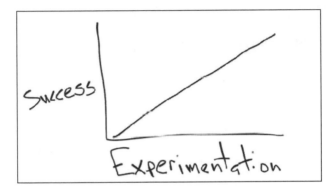

Here's the method I use:

Step One: Choose the new thing to test. It may be a food, piece of gear, exercise, what lube prevents your junk from chafing . . . whatever. Only change one variable at a time.

Step Two: Test the new variable. In many cases, this will involve going for a run or two. Pay close attention to the effects of the variable. If it is a food, how did it make you feel? Was it easy to eat? Is it something that can be carried with you?

Step Three: Decide if the variable helped or hurt, or if further experimentation is needed. If it seemed to help, adopt it as part of the training. If it hurt, abandon it. If further testing is needed, try it again.

This simple process can be used to tailor any training plan to your unique needs and abilities.

DOES BODY TYPE MATTER?

Does ultrarunning require a rail-thin emaciated body type?

Not at all! If you look at the entire field in a typical ultra, you'll find runners representing every imaginable body type. Most of the elites, both male and female, tend to be on the thinner side. As soon as you get to the next-fastest group, all bets are off. All BMIs are represented.

Losing weight generally makes you more efficient, and thus faster, but ultras are run at a slow enough speed to partially negate this effect. I'm not exactly thin myself. The last time I checked, my body fat percentage was somewhere around 15 percent. According to the experts, my "ideal" body weight is around 155 pounds. Currently I weigh around 180 pounds, but fluctuate between 170 and 195 or so. In fact, I've gotten quite a few "If *he* can run an ultra, I certainly can!" comments over the years. What can I say? I like lifting weights, eating food, and drinking beer.

Don't let your body weight or type dissuade you from running an ultra.

LISTENING TO YOUR BODY

In the barefoot running world, we *constantly* talk about the idea of listening to your body. This is a more palatable way of saying "*If it hurts, stop or do something else.*"

The same concept applies to ultrarunning. If you're doing something that causes pain, you're probably doing it wrong. Learn to listen to the signals your body gives, and then adjust accordingly.

Of course, there's a serious problem with this advice. Running really long distances hurts. A lot. Veteran ultrarunners usually refer to it as "discomfort," not "pain." Don't be fooled, *it's friggin' pain.* I'll give you some tips to deal with the pain later on, but it does leave us with the question: How do you know if it's "*I'm injured*" pain or "*This is just normal pain everybody experiences when running ultras*"?

The question is difficult to answer. Experience will teach you the difference. But what do you do in the interim? Follow these tips:

Here's my annoying disclaimer: I'm not a medical professional, and I'd recommend consulting one before doing any of this.

- **Generally speaking, muscle soreness is okay.** If you've ever lifted weights, it's that feeling you have when you first started. Never felt that? Here's a demo. Do one hundred pushups as quickly as possible. Pause to rest if needed, but the quicker the better. That burning you feel? That's usually okay. Stop reading and come back tomorrow.

(One day later)

Feel that soreness in your pecs? It's commonly referred to as DOMS, or delayed onset muscle soreness. When running, this is the soreness you'll feel for a few days after starting the activity. That pain is okay, too.

- **Sharp shooting pains are generally bad.** If it feels like someone is impaling you with a burning hot poker, you should stop. Rest until the pain subsides; seek medical attention if needed.
- **If you experience dull aches hours or a day after a workout, that could be bad.** This is especially true if the pain doesn't seem to be muscle related. Joint and bone pain are the most common areas to feel this dull ache. Rest until the pain subsides; seek medical attention if needed.
- **Some types of pain are bad.** If you experience any weird sensations or symptoms like discoloration, pain that isn't muscular, chest pain, light-headedness, numbness, abnormal swelling, fever, weight gain, or anything else abnormal, *seek immediate medical attention*. Always better to be safe than sorry. And there's always a chance the ambulance driver/nurse/doctor will be hot.

ELEMENTS OF GOOD RUNNING FORM

Good running form is one of the most neglected elements of running. For decades, we've followed a paradigm where we use various shoe designs to correct bad running form. The rise of barefoot and minimalist shoe running has created a surge of research that has progressively shifted the paradigm. We're now moving toward the idea of learning good form, then selecting shoes that don't interfere with good form. It's a subtle but significant difference.

So what is "good form"? This is a tricky issue and the research isn't nearly as conclusive as some believe. We *don't* know far more than we *do* know. What works for some may not work for others. Most seem to agree on some points, however. Here are the basics, which most people agree are the foundation for better running form:

1. **Upright posture.** Good posture is the foundation of good form. Your posture should be upright, your arms should swing freely at your sides, and your knees should remain bent throughout the gait cycle.

2. **Feet should land almost under your body.** It's common for people to overstride where their foot lands in front of their body. This is less efficient and dramatically increases the impact of running. It also reduces balance, which is critically important when trail running.

3. **Faster, shorter steps.** Your cadence, or number of steps per minute, should increase to somewhere around 180 per minute. Your stride length should also decrease. This helps ensure your feet will land under your body.

Making these adjustments will increase your efficiency and likely reduce injuries regardless of the shoes you have on your feet. While I'm a huge proponent of running barefoot and in minimalist "barefoot" shoes, they may not be appropriate for everyone in every condition. For example, barefoot and minimalist shoes suck for hundred-milers in the mountains. Even if you wear motion-control cushioned trainers with a huge raised heel, making these changes to your running form can make a dramatic difference.

Want to learn the nitty-gritty details of better running form? Check out my other wildly popular book *The Barefoot Running Book* (Plume, 2012). It consistently ranks among the top five hundred barefoot running books of all time.

RUN EFFICIENTLY

Learning good form will definitely help you become more efficient. This will allow you to run faster and longer by expending less energy. This idea can be taken further by thinking of ultra-running as an exercise in conservation. Your goal should be to use up as little energy as possible.

When I race, I try to eliminate as many wasted movements as I can. I only lift my feet high enough to clear the highest obstacle on the trail. When running up and down hills, I try to relax my muscles as much as possible and take short, easy steps. I limit my arm swing to the absolute minimum. Every wasted movement burns more precious calories.

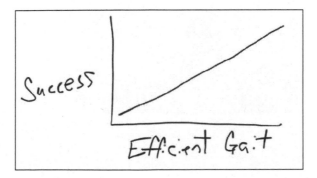

You can incorporate efficiency by actively focusing on running as smoothly as possible. Good form, as discussed earlier, will create a noticeable difference in energy expenditure. Always look for other ways to reduce movement. For example, I tie my shoes in double knots so I won't have to bend down and retie them during the race. It's a tiny detail, but many of those little details can add up.

Practicing efficient movement in every aspect of your life can help increase efficient movement when running. Back in the day I dabbled in magic. I liked to show off my prestidigitation skills in front of captive audiences at family gatherings and my classroom. Yes, I really am that dorky. Sidebar: 99 percent of the population does not appreciate a good illusion; your friends and family will probably be more annoyed than impressed when you pull out a deck of cards or a half-dollar coin. Anyway, magic is based on the idea of smooth, effortless movement. I would practice this smoothness all the time. Getting out of bed, pouring coffee, pushing a shopping cart . . . all can be an opportunity to practice smooth movements. Eventually it becomes a habit and flows over to all running-related movements.

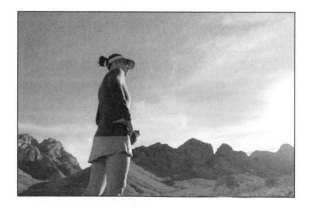

DIFFERENCE BETWEEN ROAD RUNNING GAIT AND TRAIL RUNNING GAIT

Road running and trail running require dramatically different skills. Road running utilizes the same gait for a long period of time—you're stressing a relatively small number of muscles repeatedly. Trail running requires a much more dynamic gait. Because you have to jump around the trail to avoid obstacles like rocks, roots, and water, you stress a large number of muscles in various combinations.

When road runners run trails for the first time, they're often struck by the difficulty of utilizing different muscle groups. The same phenomenon happens when trail runners run roads for the first time, though the effect isn't quite as pronounced. If you train in conditions you'll likely experience during a race, this will not be an issue. However, I would advise any runner to add at least one run per week on a different surface. Road runners should occasionally hit the trails. Trail runners should occasionally hit the road. It will dramatically enhance your ability to switch between the two.

For my first trail marathon and fifty-miler, I trained almost exclusively on roads. The trails killed me because I wasn't used to the dynamic movements. I had to walk up hills backward toward the end of those early races because my muscles simply wouldn't function properly. Over the last few years, I've shied away from road running. Whenever I run a road race, it takes much longer to recover.

UPHILL TECHNIQUE

Unless you do all your running in Florida or Nebraska, you will probably encounter the occasional hill. How should you approach the hill? Should you modify your technique? Does it depend on the surface? Are there other important variables? Let's find out.

The Basics

The single biggest mistake people make when running uphill is an elongated stride. People take steps that are too big. The longer the step you take, the more energy you'll expend over that distance. It's more efficient to take two shorter steps instead of one longer step. You can experiment with this idea by running up a flight of stairs. Hit each step on the first trip up. Then try taking two steps at a time. Then try three. Which condition was the easiest?

Posture

Posture shouldn't change from your flat-ground running gait. There's no need to lean forward or lean back. In fact, doing either will upset your balance and increase the likelihood of falling. Keep your back straight and your head up. Resist the urge to bend at the waist as this stresses the lower back.

Power Hiking

I power hike almost all steep hills in training and races over marathon distance. It's more efficient than running. The power hike is a bit of a misnomer because you're not really "powering" up the hill. The movements require very little muscle activation. Take very short (three- to twelve-inch) steps. The steeper the incline, the shorter the steps. When your foot is planted on the ground, use your gluteus muscles (butt) to lift your body up and forward over your planted foot. This motion can be assisted by straightening your knee. I like to visualize my knee moving backward to move from the bent to straight position.

Most people seem to use their quadriceps muscles (front of your thigh) to power hike, which causes premature fatigue. It's common to hear runners complain of "trashed quads." You know you're doing it right if you can climb a hill of any length without experiencing excessive burning in your quads.

Running

If the hill isn't especially steep or you're running a shorter distance, you can maintain a running gait when climbing. Like power hiking, posture doesn't change. I don't change other elements of gait except stride length and cadence. Like power hiking, I'll take shorter, faster steps instead of longer, slower steps. The same efficiency concept applies.

The muscle activation pattern is close to the same, too. I don't rely on my quads to "power" up the hill. Instead, I use my glutes to lift my body up and forward. It's a far more resilient muscle group.

Foot Placement

This lesson applies mostly to trails. When the trail gets too steep, your foot can't dorsiflex (pull your foot up toward your shin) enough to keep your heel on the ground. I always look for the flattest grades to place my feet whether I'm running or power hiking. I'll use debris like sticks, roots, and rocks as "steps." The purpose is to limit the dorsiflexion of the foot. If your foot dorsiflexes too much, it strains your calf muscles and Achilles tendon. I also try to get as much of my foot on the ground as possible for maximum traction. Slipping down the hill wastes energy. If your foot begins to slip, quickly place your other foot on the ground and shift the weight to that foot.

Picking Your Line

Like foot placement, picking your line is more of a trail running issue. Many runners just run or hike up hills with little regard for the "line," or route, they choose. Instead of just picking a random path, use the terrain to your advantage. I borrowed this technique from Jesse Scott, who used it when racing dirt bikes. Use the same "short step" technique I discussed above and pick out a line that requires the shortest steps. In other words, avoid a line that requires you to take large steps, especially if you're stepping on or over a large rock, root, or log.

Practicing

The best way to master going uphill is to practice frequently. I spent several months training with a heart rate monitor to gauge my technique. I'd climb a hill at a specific pace and measure my average heart rate. Then I'd try a slightly different technique and measure that average heart rate. I'd compare the techniques and use the one that was most efficient. I would then test that technique on some really long mountain climbs (three to six miles). If you don't live near mountains, a treadmill set on 12–15 percent grade will work. If I felt any muscle fatigue, I practiced keeping those muscles relaxed.

Using this methodology, I was able to fine-tune my technique to the point where I could climb pretty much any hill with ease. It's been a major reason I've been able to run hundred-milers on relatively low training mileage.

DOWNHILL TECHNIQUE

Running uphill was a relatively easy skill to learn. Downhill was a different story. I tried every single method I came across but nothing seemed to work. Repeatedly running downhill hurt my knees and back, and it never felt as efficient as running uphill or on flat ground. After years of experimentation, I finally stumbled upon two good techniques to assist downhill running. Both were suggested by Jesse, which were modifications of Danny Dryer's ChiRunning techniques. First, I shift my weight backward by pulling my shoulders back a little bit . . . sort of like pinching my shoulder blades together. Second, I "sit back" slightly like I'm in a chair. Since this subject is much more difficult to visualize than uphill technique, I demonstrate the idea in this YouTube video: *www.youtube.com/watch?v=oDSrUyzFPKc.*

On very steep terrain, I may utilize the "ski technique" discussed in the second part of the video. I basically mimic the back-and-forth twisting of a downhill skier negotiating moguls. It's slow but effectively allows more of the foot to come in contact with the ground, which increases control. If I start sliding, it's easier to regain control.

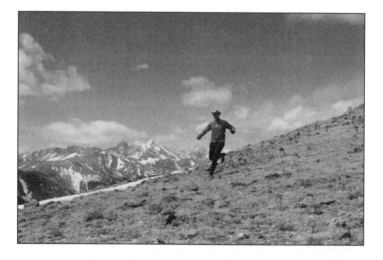

BREATHING

Breathing technique is one element of running I never considered until I was conducting a clinic in conjunction with Dr. Mark Cucuzzella at his Two Rivers Treads running store in Shepherdstown, West Virginia. He taught a deep breathing technique that involved placing one hand on your chest and the other over your belly button. When inhaling, the goal was to make your belly expand more than your chest. Look down at your hands. The hand on your chest should remain relatively stationary while the hand over your belly button should be moving in and out. This "belly breathing" helps deliver more oxygen to the blood stream.

I found this technique to be most useful when climbing hills, especially at higher altitudes. This tiny detail had a huge impact on my fatigue levels as races progressed. The technique isn't necessarily intuitive, as most of us take quick, shallow breaths (chest breathing). This is definitely a technique that requires practice during training runs.

SO HOW DO YOU GET FASTER?

Running faster is usually a function of training more. Refining technique to become more efficient, adding speedwork to your training routine, and adding hill repeats on occasion will increase your capacity for speed. (The last two are discussed later in the ultramarathon training section.)

If your goal is to get faster at running ultras, actually improving running speed isn't terribly critical. It's rare to run hard in really long races. Focusing on walking faster will shave more time off your finishes than running faster. Luckily, becoming a faster walker is much easier than becoming a fast runner. It's more about learning technique than actually improving aerobic or anaerobic conditioning.

I recommend two different workouts, each done once per week.

Workout #1: Walk as fast as you can for two or three miles. This is a sustained effort. Try to maintain as fast a pace as possible without breaking into a running gait.

Workout #2: Alternate between walking fast and running. Again, I recommend a two- to three-mile route. Start by walking a quarter mile, then run at a slow pace for a quarter mile. Repeat for the entire distance.

Since neither of these workouts are high impact, they can be added to whatever routine you're currently doing. If needed, adjust the distance. Personally I haven't found much benefit to walking more than two to three miles in one session, so it's not a workout that will grow longer with experience.

STRETCHING AND ROLLING

Should you stretch before a run? How about after? What's the deal with foam rollers and that "stick" thingy?

All of these are legitimate questions, and science doesn't really give conclusive answers. I personally do not stretch, but I occasionally use a rolling pin if I have an especially tight muscle. Instead of stretching, I prefer to warm up by doing whatever activity I'm about to do. For example, before running I walk for a few minutes and then progress to a short, slow run. For ultras, I may just start the race with a walk. I used to do extensive stretching before and after running, but I didn't see a significant benefit. It just took up more time.

I would recommend, like with everything else, experimentation. Find a good stretching or rolling routine, do it for a few weeks, and see how you feel. If it improves performance, recovery, or you find it to be enjoyable, keep at it. If it doesn't do anything for you, drop it.

Oh, and the "Stick?" It's just a ridiculously expensive rolling pin designed to separate yuppies from their hard-earned cash. Buy a five-dollar rolling pin at your local department store, then spend the rest on a race entry.

If you're especially lazy and aren't interested in stretching or rolling yet still feel tight, try taking a shot or two of Jim Beam. It may not improve performance, but it should make the subjective running experience more enjoyable.

FOOT CARE

The feet of a trail runner typically endure more punishment than road runners. The dynamic terrain, steep grades, dirt, gravel, sand, and water crossings can be brutal. Well-fitting shoes, good socks, and appropriate preventative measures can go a long way toward keeping your feet in good working condition.

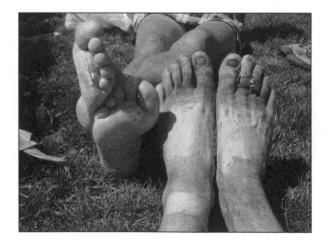

The biggest danger to your feet tends to be blisters. Knowing how blisters form is helpful for prevention. Jon VonHof's excellent book, *Fixing Your Feet,* discusses three variables needed for blisters to form: heat, moisture, and friction. In my experience, blisters can form with only one or two variables *if the conditions are severe.* The key to prevention is managing all three.

To control moisture, start with a well-ventilated shoe. Ventilation allows sweat and water from water crossings or puddles to evaporate. Moisture-wicking socks also help keep the feet relatively dry. Cotton socks generally suck for running purposes. Some people like to use various powders on their feet, but I find that they just turn to paste.

To control friction, start with shoes that fit the shape of your foot. Tie the shoes in a way that anchors the shoe to the foot to limit "sloppiness" of fit. If the shoes cannot be securely anchored, socks can be used to reduce friction. Some people even wear two thin pairs of socks. Lubrication can also be used. You should be able to determine where hot spots (friction points) occur during training runs. Lube those spots.

Heat is usually the most difficult variable to control. Ventilated shoes will help regulate foot temperature, but you're still at the mercy of the environment. Getting your feet wet is a common strategy, but it introduces the moisture variable. Besides, sweat doesn't evaporate (thus cool) in the confines of most shoes. I've used huarache sandals (à la the Tarahumara), but they present a host of other issues. When training, purposely get your feet wet to test the draining and drying properties of your shoes and socks. Keeping socks dry will usually help with cooling.

SPEEDWORK

There are a few types of runs that make up most training plans. The first I'll discuss is speedwork. As the name implies, speedwork involves running really fast. Different people have different ideas of what exactly constitutes speedwork. I'm going with a simple definition:

Speedwork can be any run where talking is extremely difficult.

Speedwork helps make you faster. There aren't too many times you'll need speed in ultras, especially your first. I recommend speedwork to prevent you from getting slower over time, so it is appropriate for new trail runners. Long-term ultrarunners who only run long, slow distances usually experience a degree of muscle atrophy and loss of speed. Occasionally running fast helps prevent that. Speedwork can also be handy if you're single and yearn to hear heavy breathing again.

Speedwork can take several forms. Some people like running repeats or laps around a track. Others like to do tempo runs, which are shorter, faster runs. I prefer running short races, like

5ks, or adding a sprinting component to my cross-training. I'm not a huge fan of fast running, so I've used some various "motivational" methods over the years.

My favorite method involved sprinting down sand hills. It was easy, fun, and made me feel *really* fast.

The best method involved an evil workout called a Tabata. The Tabata interval is named after Dr. Izumi Tabata. His team of researchers discovered doing exercise following a specific timed interval could increase anaerobic capacity and VO2 max (a measure of how efficiently your body uses oxygen to fuel muscles). It involved sprinting for 30 seconds, walking for 20, then repeating that cycle eight times. I'd rest for a few seconds, then do it again. I repeated the eight cycles six times. I threw up twice. It wouldn't have been so bad if it weren't for the Taco Bell spicy burrito I ate a few hours before.

TREADMILL TABATAS

Treadmills suck. There's no better way to put it. If I had to choose between always having to run on a treadmill and quitting running, I'd quit running. There's one notable exception: The *treadmill Tabata*. The standard interval is 20 seconds of high intensity work followed by 10 seconds of rest. Shelly and I use a treadmill adaptation. We set the treadmill at a 15 percent grade, speed anywhere from 4.5 to 7 mph, then run for 20 seconds, step off the belt to rest for 10 seconds, then repeat for a total of eight intervals. Without a doubt, it's the most difficult four minute exercise I've ever done.

The workout produces results, though. Both my finish times and climbing ability increased significantly after including treadmill Tabatas in my own routine. I usually like to add treadmill Tabatas once per week starting about three months before a goal race.

FARTLEKS

A Fartlek run is a run where your speed is going to vary for random distances. Sometimes you run fast; sometimes you run slow. The distance is usually relatively short, maybe a few miles.

You should do Fartlek runs for no other reason than the name. It's fun to say, "I'm going out to do a Fartlek!"

If you need more justification, you should do them because they train your body to make the adjustment from running fast to running slow to walking, and back. In an ultra, you'll probably make this transition several (if not many) times. This training run will help. You also get some of the benefits of speedwork without as much "vomit" danger. When you begin to reach that threshold, you just slow down.

HILL REPEATS

Hill repeats involve running up and down hills, usually at a high intensity. I love hill repeats. In my experience, it's the single most effective type of ultramarathon training. You develop strength from running uphill and speed from running downhill.

When we lived in Michigan, our hill-repeat workouts were done on an old garbage pile turned ski hill. It was like visiting Disney World and Mickey was handing out free bacon. Yes, that was sarcasm. Some people called it a "mountain" but it barely qualified as a hill. Since we didn't have too many large hills, we would do multiple repeats for each workout. Sand dunes along the pristine shore of Lake Michigan also made for a good hill-repeat workout.

Since we've been traveling around, we've had the opportunity to run up and down a lot of mountain trails. This usually results in a single run up and down without multiple repeats. Either method works.

If you live in an area that has no hills, you could get some of the same effect by running up and down the stairs of skyscrapers.

Or you could run up and down parking garages. If you have a treadmill, you can set the incline to simulate uphill running. If the treadmill has a foldable deck, you can prop up the back with a concrete block to simulate downhill running. Just don't fall.

Tip: If you are running a race that features hills, do hill repeats! As I mentioned earlier, my first trail marathon and fifty-miler were run on a fairly hilly course. I didn't do any hill repeats. It sucked. I was passed by a lady in her late sixties doing her first-ever race because I had to walk the hills backward.

THE LONG RUN

Be honest. You probably thought I skimped on the last few explanations of the other training runs. It's because most ultrarunners don't do them. They spend most of their time and energy focusing on the centerpiece of every training plan: the long run.

Well, except for Crossfit Endurance. If that was your training run selection, go ahead and skip this part. CFE frowns on the logic behind the long, slow run so you never have the opportunity to learn the subtle nuances of covering long distances. Should you decide to choose CFE as your primary training plan, be ready to face a lot of unknowns such as reaching the fifty-mile mark and having your ass crack get severely chafed, then the cheeks fusing together as they heal. It really happens. Google it.

Okay, where was I? Oh yeah, the long run. The long run serves two purposes:

First, it trains your body to deal with the rigors of running long distances. You accomplish this by increasing your long run distance gradually over time. It strengthens your muscles, tendons, ligaments, bones, endocrine system, and any other bodily systems that are stressed over long distances.

Second, it allows you to experiment in conditions that are at least somewhat similar to race conditions. How is that water bottle going to feel after twenty-four miles? Will those packets of spaghetti-flavored Gu still taste good after eight hours of running? Can you bend over to tie your shoes after thirty miles? How about needing to squat to drop a deuce? You can't test these variables without the long run.

Long runs can take on a few different flavors. You could do one single long, continuous run. You could do two shorter runs over two days. You could do five or six shorter runs over the course of one day. Different plans will use one of the different flavors. Personally, I like to do all three, though I use the first more than the last two.

When I design my own plans, I like to schedule a run that is long enough for me to develop an "ultra hurt." I want to experience the point where the pain starts getting annoying, the point where I have to start actively dealing with it. This usually comes at about the twenty-five- to thirty-mile mark.

The longest training run I've ever done is the infamous Kal-Haven double crossing in southwest Michigan. Jesse Scott, Mark Robillard, and I set out on a sixty-eight mile out-and-back on a thirty-four mile rails-to-trails path. It sucked. We had a friend, Tony Schaub, riding a bike to carry some of our gear, but it did little to dampen the extreme beating our bodies took.

It definitely crossed the "this run is too long to produce a positive training effect, and will likely just hurt us" threshold. I ran a hundred-miler three weeks later and definitely suffered more than I should have. It set me up for a serious case of overtraining, which shelved me for months.

The lesson: Long training runs are important learning tools. *Really* long training runs are stupid.

CROSS-TRAINING

We're preparing to run a race. As such, we should run a lot. Right?

Not always. Many new ultrarunners make the mistake of focusing entirely on running and ignoring any other form of exercise.

The problem?

If you do nothing but run, you'll likely develop muscle imbalances, which may lead to injury. Cross-training can increase flexibility, muscle endurance, and recovery. It will also prepare your body for some of the unexpected elements of ultras. For example, the weight training I do allows me to carry my water bottle for the duration of races. That twenty-ounce bottle of water gets quite heavy after a hundred miles.

So what are the options? Pretty much any nonrunning exercise will be effective cross-training. Here are some ideas:

- Mountain biking
- Yoga
- Rowing
- Unicycling (thanks Rob Youngren)
- Weight training
- Competing in the Lumberjack Games
- Testing the entire Kama Sutra
- Swimming
- MMA training

If you want one specific recommendation, I suggest functional fitness–high intensity interval training. It combines exercises that utilize a wide variety of muscle groups with workout formats that make you sweat. A lot.

Crossfit is usually viewed as a form of functional fitness. P90X is another popular program. Both are rather intense and would probably lead to overtraining and injury if done in conjunction with a full running program. Use their workouts but limit them to two or three per week. If I were to give a specific recommendation, I'd suggest Pete Kemme's workouts, which can be found at *www.kemmefitness.com*. His workouts range from mild to extreme, so they appeal to beginners, experts, and everyone in between. One of his more famous workouts involved doing a burpee then leaping forward . . . for a mile. He's also fond of using homemade gym equipment like slosh tubes, doing weird "animal walks" up and down stairs, and creating a thousand ways to do a pushup. Pete's crazy workouts helped me finish all of my hundred-milers. Don't be afraid to mix it up. Any physical activity other than running will help train you for ultras.

DIET IN GENERAL

Religion, abortion, immigration policy . . . none of these controversial topics seem to elicit the sheer passion on social media as diet philosophy. Vegans, Paleo folks, fruitarians, and organic fanatics are a passionate bunch. The supposed supporting evidence for various diet philosophies makes this a tricky issue. Pretty much every popular diet will claim to be supported by science. In reality, there may only be a handful of small studies supporting it—the rest is nothing more than opinion and propaganda from "professionals" who sell books and product related to the diet.

The simple fact that humans, throughout history and around the world today, are able to survive on a wide variety of diets should dispel the idea that there's one universal "best" diet. Furthermore, suggesting there's one ideal diet for all disregards the needs of different individuals. What's good for me won't necessarily be good for you. We like to ignore the obvious, though.

So how should we determine our diet? I like to use a really simple philosophy based on experimentation and common sense. Let's call it the "moderation and variation" diet. Eat whatever you want as long as it's done in moderation (don't eat too much of one single food) and variation (eat lots of different foods). This will ensure we get all the necessary nutrients needed to sustain life. Also, eat roughly the same number of calories you burn. If one single food seems to have a negative effect, cut it from your diet.

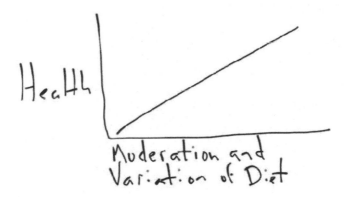

I utilize this diet by shopping mostly around the perimeter of my grocery stores where produce, dairy, eggs, and meats can be found. I tend to buy whatever happens to be on sale, which assures a great deal of variety. I buy less prepared, processed foods because they tend to have a higher calorie count than fresh, whole foods. Shelly and I also enjoy cooking, and the fresh ingredients taste better.

Remember one simple fact: *If you're overweight, it's because you're eating and drinking too much.* Many people make the mistake of simply *adding* "healthy" food to their diet, which just adds more calories. Cutting out a few high-calorie/low-satisfaction foods and drinks can make a dramatic difference in achieving and maintaining a healthy body weight.

SUPPLEMENTS

The dietary supplement industry sells around 23 billion dollars worth of products each year. I've known runners who swear by a wide variety of supplements, the most common of which seem to be:

- Iron
- Fish oil
- Creatine
- Calcium
- Multivitamins

The science behind any supplements tends to be somewhat shady. Yes, humans have specific vitamin and mineral needs. Yes, some of us may be deficient *if we don't eat a balanced diet.* Almost all of us will be perfectly fine as long as we keep things interesting. As I discussed above, there should be no need for dietary supplements if we eat a lot of different-colored food from the perimeter of the grocery store. Moderation and variation provide all we need. Since extra vitamins are expelled from the body, it has been said that a person could make a fortune mining the vitamins from the urine of Americans. Save the money you'd spend on supplements for future race fees or that dream "running" vacation to Rocky Mountain National Park.

FOOD BEFORE A RUN

Through extensive experimentation, I've managed to find a handful of foods that work well as a pre-run meal. The criteria is straightforward: the food has to be easy to digest and give me plenty of energy that will last for a relatively long time, yet still be relatively "digestible."

My preferred foods, in order of preference, are Pop Tarts (frosted strawberry, the only *real* Pop Tart flavor), muffins, and miniature donuts. As you can tell, I'm a fan of sweet pastries.

To figure out which foods work best for you, test a different food before each run. I would recommend giving a food at least two opportunities, as results can be influenced by other factors.

Some other popular foods include fruit, oatmeal, breakfast cereal, pancakes, French toast, or anything from the breakfast menu at McDonald's. There are some foods to avoid, namely spicy foods. Good rule of thumb: if it's hot going in, it's going to be hotter going out. The "burning ring of fire" atomic anal sphincter can be a major distraction.

FOOD DURING A RUN

Fueling during a run can be difficult logistically, so I would recommend taking two approaches:

1. **Train using food typically found at ultra aid stations, like candy, chips, boiled potatoes, cookies, soda, peanut butter and jelly sandwiches, or any specific food a goal race advertises**. This will allow you to use aid stations for fueling if necessary. I prefer to use my own food, but I have run into situations when it wasn't available. Learning to fuel off what is available can solve a lot of potential problems.

2. **Find foods that work well for you**. This includes foods that are easy to carry, can be stuffed in drop bags, or can be carried by your crew. Since many ultras are run far from civilization, non perishable foods that require little or no preparation are ideal. Also, your palate will change throughout a race. What tastes good at mile five probably won't taste good at mile thirty-five or mile ninety-five. Test different foods at different distances. Don't overdo

it, though. It is possible to develop a taste aversion to a particular food if you train with it too much. If that happens, the food will be useless during a race. I made this mistake with gels. I used them all the time when training and got to the point where I couldn't stomach them later in races. The solution was to completely abstain from gels for about a year.

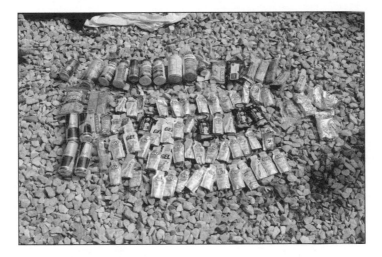

A selection of ultra food I used for the Grindstone 100.

FOOD AFTER A RUN

"Recovery" food has become a bit of an interesting topic in the running world. Conventional wisdom that existed for decades suggested eating a carbohydrate-rich meal within ninety minutes of running to replace the carbs lost during the run. A few runners have been advocating different approaches ranging from high protein (the Paleo crowd) to fruits (fruitarians) to fasting (supermodels).

In my own experimentation, I found virtually no effect with any of these approaches. While some are backed by a study or two, no approach really accounts for the variability that exists in humans. My logical solution: *eat based on cravings*. If you're hungry, eat; if not, don't. If steak sounds good, eat steak. If ice cream sandwiches sound good, eat ice cream sandwiches. Same deal with beer, avocados, or Cheerios.

Pay attention to the effects of various foods. Eventually you will probably notice a pattern. Certain foods will make you feel better the rest of the day. Some foods may help you on your next run. When you find something that works, stick with it.

WHAT TO DRINK

When it comes to hydration, there are a ton of usable options. I'll run down the list in order of relative popularity.

- **Sports drinks:** This includes products like Gatorade, Heed, Nuun, GU Brew, etc. Most sports drinks provide electrolytes, which are lost via sweat. Most also contain varying amounts of calories, which help you stay fueled. In most races, sports drinks are my preferred option, though I sometimes switch to water toward the end. The sweetness of sports drinks sometimes makes me nauseous.
- **Water:** Many people prefer good ole water during a race. Water doesn't provide electrolytes or calories, but is palatable throughout a race.
- **Soda:** Not many people use soda, but it does contain calories and some sodium. The carbonation can make it more palatable. If the soda is caffeinated, it may cause a slight diuretic effect. I'll toss energy drinks into this category, too, though the high caffeine levels make it

impractical for a primary hydration strategy. Unless you're a crack addict.

- **Juice:** Juice is actually a pretty good option and was more popular before the widespread use of sports drinks. It tends to be relatively high in caloric content, but also has a heavy flavor.

- **Beer/ Wine/other Alcohol:** I've experimented with both beer and wine, and once did an unfortunate "tequila run." The result of all three was roughly the same: it sucked. The bitterness of beer seemed to become enhanced the longer I ran, which ruled out any good beer. I tried drinking beers like Michelob Ultra, but I had a hard time distinguishing it from water. Wine was okay, but I needed to drink too much to remain relatively well hydrated. Drunkenness inhibits trail running. Go figure.

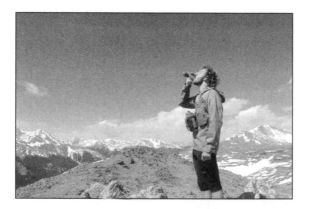

Jesse Scott enjoying a high altitude energy drink.

FOOD

Running burns energy . . . *a lot* of energy. Most people burn somewhere around 110 to 130 calories per mile traveled. Over the course of an ultra or long trail run, that adds up to at least tens of thousands of calories. As I prepare for an ultra, I like to get an idea of how much food I will need to consume and I like to simplify this process as much as possible.

Before starting the process, let's look at a few principles. Your body can use two primary fuel sources: carbohydrates and fat. Carbs burn quickly and efficiently. Fat burns slowly. If you're running fast, your body will burn carbs. The slower you run, the more fat your body uses as fuel. The "crashing" feeling you get is the result of making the switch from carb burning to fat burning.

You have a limited supply of carbs available at any given time, but you have a *huge* supply of fat. If you want to burn carbs, you need to constantly replace them by consuming calories during the run. This will allow you to run faster. You could get by without eating anything and rely on your fat stores, but you would have to keep intensity to a minimum. It's like the difference between throwing a piece of newspaper on a fire versus a giant oak log: the paper burns quickly with a huge flame while the log burns longer with a much less intense flame.

Through training, I know I can run about eighteen miles before my carbohydrate supply is exhausted. At that point, my body switches to fat-burning mode—I slow down considerably and experience a crash. I can calculate a ballpark estimate of the carbs I have to consume during the run to avoid that crash by subtracting 18 from the total miles of the race, then multiplying that number by 100.

50 miles – 18 miles = 32 miles
32 x 100 = 3,200 calories needed during the run to avoid the crash

During a fifty-miler, I know I have to consume approximately 3,200 calories. This is where it gets a little tricky. Most people can only digest about 200–300 calories per hour. Let's assume you can process 250 calories per hour. If you're running at a twelve-minute/mile pace (for a ten-hour finish), you could consume 2,500 calories during that ten-hour race. Since you need 3,200 calories, you won't be able to consume enough to avoid a crash.

The problem becomes more pronounced with longer races. How about a hundred-miler?

100 miles – 18 miles = 82
82 x 100 = 8,200 calories needed during the run to avoid the crash

This is what I do to remedy the situation:

- **Train to eat.** I've managed to get to the point where I can comfortably eat up to 500 calories per hour when running, which allows me to keep fueling throughout most races.
- **Train to burn fat.** This is the idea behind the Maffetone method discussed at various points throughout the book. This is also the reason I occasionally do long runs after fasting for 24 hours.
- **Start consuming calories from the beginning of a race.** The longer you wait, the less opportunity you have to stay ahead of the carb game.
- **Find foods that are palatable even after running long distances.** I have at least four "backup foods" in case the aid station foods aren't cutting it.
- **Know what the "crash" feels like.** When it starts to hit, slow down and consume something sweet.

TAKING THE BAREFOOT THING TOO FAR

I was generally happy with my 2006 fifty-miler finish. Still, I thought I probably could have done a little better. I hadn't quite hit my "overresearch then endlessly experiment" phase yet, so I followed a lot of bad advice. First, I used a modified marathon plan, which consisted of slow runs of varying lengths. I spent too much time worrying about stupid useless crap (like pace charts to assure I'd finish in my goal time), and less time worrying about important stuff (could I really eat maple syrup and gummi worms for fifty miles?).

That winter, I scoured the web, read forums and race reports, subscribed to *Ultrarunning* magazine, and purchased *Running Through the Wall*, *A Step Beyond*, and *Lore of Running*. I was determined to get faster, damn it!

The intensive reading led me to an important conclusion: *there really was no single "right" answer.* Pretty much every variable associated with running ultras could be manipulated in a way to help some of the people some of the time, but never all of the people all of the time. Even a seemingly simple question like

"How many weekly miles should I run in training?" was met with a wide range of success stories. Some people ran one hundred fifty miles or more. Others barely ran twenty. At this stage of my ultra "career," I opted to choose the advice that seemed to be the most popular.

My biggest issue involved shoes. Since I was training exclusively barefoot, it was impossible to run in shoes other than my crappy-ass aqua socks. I tried going back to normal running shoes, but the cushioning and raised heel messed up my gait. I could run the race in the aqua socks again, but the fit was terrible and they were ridiculously hot. I made a decision to attempt the run barefoot.

I ran a few shorter road races to test out the barefootedness, including a small local five-kilometer race. I was standing at the start line when the race director gave a short speech. Apparently, the proceeds for the race were going to an organization that provided shoes for needy children. Everyone around me in the starting gate had a good chuckle. That particular race went well; I actually finished first in my age group. That may have been the only time that's happened.

The rest of the training for ultra number two went well, though having two small babies made it difficult at times. Like the summer before, I was relegated to night running. I didn't do nearly enough running on trails the previous year, so I added night trail runs that included both stairs and hills. I'm slightly ashamed to admit it was scary running through wooded trails alone in the darkness. Just as I was conquering my fear, I experienced a "Blair Witch" event.

I was running alone in a large wooded park on a cloudy, moonless night. My flashlight batteries were weak at the beginning of the run, but I had a backup headlamp. I reached the halfway point on the trail, which was about a mile and a half from any sort of civilization (and light source), when the flashlight died. I fumbled around in my hydration pack until I found my headlamp. I felt the on/off button. *Click.* Nothing.

After a few seconds of confusion, I suddenly remembered I had used the headlamp batteries for our daughter's mobile over her crib. One night she couldn't fall asleep. The mobile usually comforted her, but the batteries had died. In desperation, I used the ones from my headlamp and forgot to replace them. Oops.

I hadn't run the trails enough to know the precise route back to my car. Besides, I could barely discern the leaf-covered trails from the surrounding forest floor. I had a mild panic attack as I realized I only had two choices: sit in this spot in complete darkness for the four or so hours until sunrise, or wander aimlessly in the dark in the hopes I'd reach my car. Naturally, I chose the latter.

I started in the direction I thought I had come from. I would identify a tree a few feet away in the direction I was trying to travel, stumble to it, then find another tree that was in line with the tree I just left. Each time, I'd have to stop and strain to see each tree. At first, the pitch-black world was quiet, but it didn't take long before I started hearing noises. There were rustling leaves, snapping twigs, and occasionally something would fly near my head.

Logically, I knew there were very few dangerous animals in Michigan. In fact, domestic dogs were probably the biggest possible threat. Unfortunately, logic doesn't turn off the fear response. I managed to calm myself down to an extent . . . until I heard a sudden crashing about ten feet away.

I'm pretty sure I screamed like a little girl. I know I peed a little.

Needless to say, the experience was traumatic enough to make me give up trail running forever . . . if I still wasn't very far away from my car. My body could only maintain the extreme fear response for so long before exhaustion set in. I had two more "crashing" events that night, but was too tired to react. I had unwittingly used "flooding," a psychological process of eradicating phobias, to overcome my fear of the nighttime forest trails.

Somehow, I managed to keep moving in the right direction. After about an hour, I miraculously found the parking lot and drove home. After this experience, I no longer feared running on trails at night. I also developed an obsessive need to carry at least one extra light and two sets of spare batteries.

By the time the race rolled around that fall, I was prepared. I was confident I could easily shave an hour or more off my ten-and-a-half-hour finish the previous year. I knew the course, I had done the training, and I brought the right gear. I was going to kick ass!

The race pretty much went according to plan. I started a little too fast, but settled into an appropriate pace. My barefootedness was the topic of conversation with each runner I passed. As the race progressed, my confidence soared. Around mile thirty-five or so, I was on pace for a finish somewhere in the ballpark of nine and a half hours. I was mentally calculating my finish time when I looked at my watch, which made me miss the tree root protruding from the ground.

Whack!

I face-planted hard. It took a second to realize what happened. I must have tripped on something. I looked back and saw the large root. That's when the pain hit. At that point, it was the worst physical pain I had ever experienced. It felt as if my toes had been smashed by a tiny elf swinging a giant hammer. The pain was a combination of intense throbbing and searing heat.

I looked at the afflicted foot. The pinky toe on my right foot was swollen and had turned bright red. Stupidly, I immediately stood up and tried to continue running. I took two steps, vomited a few times, took a few more steps past the pool of partially digested gummi bears and taters, and passed out.

I'm pretty sure I was only out for a second or two. I was on the ground. I rolled to my back, a gentle breeze swaying the treetops high above, and contemplated my situation. The pain hadn't subsided at all and it I was at least a few miles from the next aid station. I didn't see any other runners on the trail—I had no choice but to continue on.

I looked at my foot again; my toe was now turning a deep shade of purple. I used a nearby tree to help stabilize myself as I tentatively stood up again. I felt light-headed but didn't pass out. I took a step, then another. My foot hurt something fierce, but it didn't hurt worse when walking. I started hobbling down the trail toward the next aid station.

After about a half mile, I started to get impatient. I couldn't block out the pain and just wanted to get back to Shelly at the start/finish line, so I sped up to a fast walk. It felt the same. I started running. There was no additional pain. The toe hurt just as much running as it did if I were lying down.

By the time I got to the aid station, I was close to my original pace. I must have been drunk on endorphins because I decided against telling the aid station workers about my fall. I had less than fifteen miles to go and was confident I could endure the pain. There was a chance they wouldn't let me continue, so I tried my best to give a weak smile, ate a bit, refilled my water bottle, and headed back out.

It was a long, slow journey to the finish. The pain never really subsided and I continually regretted not dropping at that first post-injury aid station. Regardless, I made it to the finish and I was incredibly relieved as I staggered across the line. My time? Still well over ten hours. I only beat my previous year's time by about ten minutes. It was hardly the dominating showing I expected, but it would fuel my desire to keep trying to master this stupid sport. Over the next few months, I'd manage to delude myself into thinking a) barefoot running and ultras really was a good combination, and b) I was ready to tackle a hundred-miler.

SECTION 3:
TRAIL RUNNING ISSUES

Trail running introduces quite a few variables you rarely find on the roads and sidewalks of suburbia. This section will cover as many as possible.

MUD

The Elements

Running through mud can be problematic for a few reasons: it may be slippery, it could clog the tread on your shoes, and if it's deep enough, you could get stuck. Worse, the mud could suck your shoes off your feet. If you're running a long race, the mud can infiltrate your shoe, and, if the mud dries inside your shoe, it leaves a gritty, abrasive mess.

Despite all of these drawbacks, mud is pretty damn fun. I only avoid mud if there's a potential to disrupt my race goals. Otherwise, I just bomb through it with a smile on my face.

Not all mud is the same, though. Some types of mud are worse than other types. A basic familiarity with mud properties can be very helpful. Here are some basics:

- **Know the local soil.** If an area has a lot of clay content, the mud will be exceedingly slippery and sticky. I try to avoid this mud on long runs or longish races. If you're running in an area with rich soil and lots of lush plants and trees, mud is usually thick. This mud usually isn't too bad as long as the mud holes aren't too deep. The shade from trees slows drying time, so mud holes may be rather deep. If the area has sandy soil, mud is usually thin and gritty. I almost always run through this stuff.

- **Know what reflectivity indicates.** Wet mud with a *shiny appearance* is fresh. And wet. And usually deep. A *dull surface* indicates mud that is drying. The dull surface is almost always safe to run over.

- **Know what's under the mud.** Mud may be covering sharp rocks (which is why it's not a good idea to run barefoot on some muddy trails), ruts from vehicle tires, hoof prints from cattle, etc. When your foot hits the mud, your brain registers it as a flat surface and proceeds to shift all your weight on that foot. As you sink through the mud, the uneven underlying surface could cause serious injuries like ankle sprains. Worse, sharp rocks may be hidden. As the foot slips, the rocks may slice your foot to shreds. My friend Nate Wolfe ran an entire race barefoot in these conditions—the result wasn't pretty.

Trail erosion can also be a concern. In some areas such as the trails surrounding Boise, Idaho, trail running on muddy trails is prohibited because it speeds erosion. In other areas like the Colorado Rockies, runners are usually encouraged to stay on muddy trails to prevent damage to the plants along them. In the Midwest, it's common to leave the trail to bypass mud holes. Be familiar with your area's rules and customs.

Shoe choice in muddy conditions is an important consideration. A cleated sole usually helps, but the cleats have to be far enough apart to prevent mud from caking between the knobs. Also, a shoe that drains well is useful. If water and mud enter the shoe, you want a mechanism in place to allow the mud and water to escape. Newbies sometimes experiment with waterproof shoes. In my experience, anything that keeps water out also keeps it in. Since mud and water easily flow over the top of the shoe, waterproof shoes are more or less useless.

SNOW AND ICE

Snow and ice introduce many of the same concerns as mud. Slipping is the greatest danger, followed by wet feet. Like mud, snow composition changes based on environmental conditions. Snow may be wet and "packy," powdery, or packed down and frozen. Each condition presents unique challenges.

- **Wet snow:** Wet snow causes everything to get wet, which usually equates to "cold." I treat this snow much like mud. It's slippery. Unless it's compressed (like on a well-used trail), it is difficult to run through due to resistance.
- **Powder:** Since the moisture content of powdery snow is low, it doesn't drench shoes and clothing. It also doesn't provide much resistance when running through deep sections. The greatest problem is with vision: powdery snow obscures the underlying surface. Since the snow is so thin, the layer that's compressed under foot does little to buffer hidden objects.

- **Hard-packed snow:** There's a fine line between compressed, hard-packed snow and ice. Functionally, they present the same problem: slipperiness. If the surface is flat, good running form should prevent most slips because your feet will always land under your center of gravity. If the surface isn't flat, like hills or cambered surfaces, shortening your stride can help prevent falling.

If you live in a cold climate, be careful with ice-covered surfaces. As a general rule of thumb, you should never attempt to cross ice thinner than about two inches. Since most runners don't carry ice-boring tools, a stick can be used to test ice—try driving it through the ice. If it breaks through, don't cross, if the ice cracks, it's probably not strong enough to support your body weight. If it doesn't crack, it should be safe to cross.

Still water freezes faster than flowing water. As such, lakes and ponds are generally safer to cross than rivers or streams. Wind also affects freezing water. In windy conditions, the churning water won't freeze as quickly as still water.

In the event you fall through ice, don't panic. Don't remove clothing as it traps air and aids in floatation. Turn toward the direction you came from, reach your arms across the ice, and kick your legs and crawl with your arms to "swim" out of the hole. Once you get out, roll to the edge of the shore. Rolling distributes more weight than walking or crawling, which will help prevent breaking through again. Get out of the cold as soon as possible since hypothermia sets in quickly. Build a fire if needed. If clothing is damp, dry it out. Wet T-shirts may be desirable for spring break in Cancun or Lake Havasu, but they can be deadly in the frozen wilderness.

WATER CROSSINGS

Trail runners occasionally encounter water crossings. These may range from a trickle of a stream to a raging river. Knowing some properties of flowing water will help you determine if a crossing is safe and what technique should be used.

Small jumpable crossings

If the crossing is small enough, just jump over it. Make sure the footing on either bank is adequate for pushing off and landing. If there's mud, use caution. Shiny mud is slippery mud. If other runners have already jumped across, it may be best to move a few feet up or downstream.

Moderate crossings that cannot be jumped over

For larger streams, you may have to hop on rocks or logs to cross, or just step in the stream. Footing is the most important consideration. It's usually best to stop, assess the options, then cross cautiously. If it is possible to hop across using rocks or logs, make sure the footing is good. Wet rocks and logs will be slippery, smaller rocks may wobble, and old logs may be rotten. Any of these could be covered with algae, moss, or other such slimy substances. If possible, test each step before fully committing all of your body weight. If the footing is questionable, just step *in* the stream. A wet foot is better than slipping and falling.

Crossings that require you to get wet

These crossings range from wide streams to rivers. If you encounter such a crossing, assess the safety of it. The speed of the current is a major consideration. The faster the current, the more dangerous the crossing. Debris like sticks, logs, and plant matter are good indicators of flow rate.

Also consider the footing in the stream or river. Mud may cause you to sink, lose a shoe, or get stuck; sharp rocks could cause foot injuries; and flat rocks could be slippery.

Knowing the properties of streams and rivers can help determine a safe crossing point. The goal is to find the shallowest crossing, which is almost always found in straight, wide sections. The deepest areas of flowing bodies of water are found on the *outer* edge of bends. Anything more than knee-deep can easily sweep you off your feet. Also consider the entry and exit points. Make sure you will be able to safely enter and exit the water.

When crossing, face toward the current. Maintain balance by shuffling your feet—using a stick as a pole will help maintain balance. If you get swept off your feet, keep your head facing upstream and swim toward the closest shore.

If you're part of a group and the crossing is especially dangerous, you can utilize the "linked-arm" technique. By linking arms and using the technique described above, you can help each other maintain balance as you cross. Imagine the "We are the World" folks. Now imagine we throw them into a wild river.

A note about parasites

In some delicate ecosystems, crossing multiple streams should be avoided due to invasive species transmission. Crossing one stream will pick up some tiny travelers, which can then be deposited in another stream. This probably isn't a concern unless you're running very long distances. If you *are* crossing multiple streams and there's a concern with cross-contamination, change your shoes between crossings or use a disinfecting agent. In my experience, this is only a concern in high mountain zones where people seem to care about the preservation of the local ecology. In many areas, we just rely on toxic waste runoff from factories to kill invasive species.

ALTITUDE

Some of the world's best trails are found in mountains. The spectacular scenery, deep blue skies, and solitude are nothing short of amazing. Unfortunately, mountain running has a serious drawback: thin air. The higher the altitude, the lower the oxygen content of the air we breathe. The thinner the air, the more problems humans develop.

Altitude sickness has a few common symptoms including breathlessness, nausea, dizziness, headaches, loss of appetite, trouble sleeping, and muscle weakness. It *is* possible to die from altitude sickness (via pulmonary or cerebral edema).

Altitude sickness is not necessarily universal; it only affects a certain percentage of the population. There are no reliable predictors to determine susceptibility other than a lack of acclimation. People who live at or near sea level and then venture to high altitudes experience the problems.

Symptoms typically begin around 5,000 to 6,000 feet up to about 8,000 feet. The higher the altitude, the more severe the symptoms.

Prevention

The best way to prevent altitude sickness is acclimation, which involves spending time at altitude. Spending several weeks at the desired altitude will usually prevent most problems. Slowly increasing the ascent can also help. For example, if you're racing at 12,000 feet, spend a few days at 6,000 feet, then 8,000, then 10,000 feet. If that's not possible, running within twenty-four hours of arrival at altitude is usually desirable.

Staying well-hydrated can also prevent altitude sickness symptoms. Drink lots of water and avoid diuretics like caffeine and alcohol. That last one is worth repeating: limit alcohol! We frequently went from low to high altitudes when traveling and the effects of alcohol were definitely enhanced when going low to high. I distinctly remember getting quite drunk from a few light beers then experiencing pretty bad hangovers for the first few days in the mountains.

Some drugs such as acetazolamide, dexamethasone, sumatriptan, and Myo-inositol trispyrophosphate (ITPP) may help treat or even prevent symptoms. However, like most drugs, they may have undesirable side effects that could inhibit athletic performance. There are products that supposedly ease acclimation problems, but I'd recommend a skeptical approach. Self-experimentation with and without supplements should be enough to assess the validity of any marketing claims.

NIGHT RUNNING

Running at night is a useful skill to develop. Many ultras have some degree of night running. Checking the start time and cutoff time of your race, then checking the morning and evening civil twilight times, is always a good idea. Civil twilight is the point where the sun is 6 degrees below the horizon. In most cases, this is the time when it is possible to see your surroundings without a flashlight.

Running at night is relatively straightforward; just plan a few runs after dark. If I'm running a race that requires running through the night, I'll plan two types of runs: a very late run and a very early run. The late run usually starts around 10 p.m. and ends around 2 a.m. The early morning run starts around 2 a.m. and ends around 6 p.m. The idea is to acclimate your body to running during the hours you'd normally be sleeping.

If you will be using an artificial light, most people use either a handheld flashlight or a headlamp. I would recommend carrying both. Use the flashlight as the primary light source and the headlamp as a backup. Since the flashlight can be carried near the waist, it will cast longer shadows on the trail. This makes it easier to identify and avoid obstacles like rocks, roots, and cobras. The headlamp is useful if you need hands-free light, like for eating at aid stations or pooping.

Some ultrarunners strap a headlamp to their chest or waist. I've tried this method but the light bounced too much. It also limits the ability to look to the side without having to move your entire body. Still, it may be a worthwhile experiment.

POOPING

"What happens when I have to . . . you know, take a number two?"

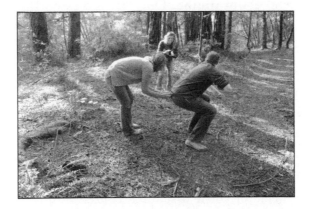

Shelly and Krista Cavender watching Pablo Paster demonstrating a decent poop squat.

I am a little surprised this question does not come up more often. Here's the situation: You're thirty miles into a fifty-mile run and surrounded by nothing but untamed wilderness.

You have to drop a deuce. Since there are no Porta Potties for another twenty miles, you are left with no choice but to drop drawers and let loose.

I always assume everyone has the benefit of being raised in the sticks and I sometimes forget my suburbanite friends have probably never had the opportunity to hone their wilderness bowel movement skills. I am also somewhat surprised at the amount of anxiety some people feel at the thought of dropping a deuce outside the friendly confines of the vertical plastic coffins we call Pora Potties neatly lined up at the start line of races.

My first bit of advice: *practice*. Don't wait until race day to attempt a torpedo launch in the woods. Next time you're out on the trails, find a secluded spot and give it a go. So how do you actually go about pooping in the wilderness?

1. **It's all about timing.** Don't try too early. The squatting position you'll adopt is difficult to maintain for more than a minute or two.
2. **Get off the trail.** Twenty feet is usually the minimum. Stay away from water sources. If possible, move out of the line of sight and downwind of others—it's the courteous thing to do.
3. **Secure your wiping material beforehand.** Any paper will do, as will a bandana or sock. If those items aren't available or you're a staunch conservationist, try leaves, pine cones, sticks, or flat rocks.
4. **If possible, dig a small six-inch by six-inch hole, three to four inches deep.** This will be the poo hole.
5. **When pulling down your pants, make sure they're clear of the path the poo will take from butt to ground.**

It's the same deal with shoes. You don't want to be sideswiped by a butt nugget.

6. **When squatting, use trees or logs for support if needed.** Practice a variety of positions so you will be prepared for a variety of situations.

7. **Drop the deuce.**

8. **DON'T STAND UP RIGHT AWAY!** It will clench your cheeks together, which increases the required wiping.

9. **After the wiping is done, cover the poo with a little dirt, then mix it up.** This aids the decomposition process.

10. **Cover the poo/dirt mixture to prevent others from stepping in it.** I also like to disguise the hole to maintain that "undisturbed nature" look.

Here are some additional pointers:

- When actually squatting, it can be beneficial to hold your cheeks apart. Sadly, I have to credit MTV's *The Real World* for this tip.

- Keeping a small piece of biodegradable toilet paper or wet wipes in your pocket can help with the final cleanup procedure.

- When choosing a location to squat, most people simply wander a fair distance from the trail. Make sure you don't inadvertently walk too close to a different trail or road.

- Know what the local poisonous plants are . . . don't squat in them. I knew an ultrarunner who squatted in some poison oak. Damn near rectum!

- Avoid plants with thorns, too.

- Same deal with bees.

THERMOREGULATION

This issue could affect road runners also, but the possible remoteness of trail running makes it significantly more dangerous for trail runners. Early in 2012 I wrote a post about some difficulties I had in hot, dry weather. I theorized about the role a moisture-wicking shirt played in three crappy runs over a period of several months. After reading the comments from my audience and doing a little research, I came to an obvious conclusion: *moisture-wicking clothing does more harm than good for runners in hot, dry weather.*

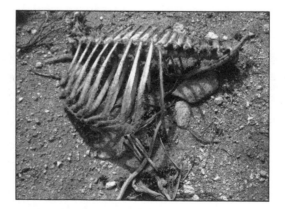

The reasoning is simple: the mechanism of drawing moisture away from the skin thwarts the process of evaporative cooling of sweat. In other words, the wicking of the moisture means the sweat evaporates on the surface of the shirt, not your skin, so you're robbing your body of one of the primary cooling mechanisms used to reduce your core body temperature.

The marketing material from several moisture wicking companies confirms this. They are very guarded about saying the fabric cools you down in heat. Instead, they tend to use statements like "the fabric makes you feel more comfortable." Indeed, moisture wicking fabrics are great . . . when you're not generating a ton of heat via exercise.

My rule of thumb: I'm only using moisture-wicking fabric in cold weather or in warmer weather when my activity level is low enough where body temps can be maintained without the sweating mechanism. If I am running in hot weather, I'm going with loose-fitting white cotton or no shirt at all.

Thermoregulation: My Missing Link

I did a lot of experimenting with perceived body temperature and how it made me feel. I believe my problems at Bighorn in 2012, a disastrous Boulder to Nederland, Colorado, run in 2012, and the 2011–2012 Across the Years race were all caused by overheating.

During each of those events, I knew heat was the problem . . . indirectly. I assumed I wasn't drinking enough (dehydration) or I wasn't taking enough electrolyte supplementation (hyponatremia). These are the two often-quoted causes of the symptoms I was experiencing. In fact, most runners recommended either drinking more or taking more electrolytes.

The feelings I was having weren't quite right, though. In training, I had purposely run to a point of dehydration. Early in my running "career," I also experienced the early signs of hyponatremia. Neither of these feelings were quite the same. There was some other variable I was missing.

That variable was a rising core body temperature.

Generally I'm a pretty good hot weather runner. I can tolerate heat far better than cold. In the humid Midwest, I used to run on the hottest of days with no issues at all. I didn't experience this problem until I started running in hot, *dry* weather . . . and then only when wearing moisture-wicking shirts.

As I explained previously, the moisture-wicking material apparently caused my core temperature to rise faster than my sweating mechanism (and passive heat-dissipation methods) could get rid of the excess. The result was extreme fatigue, dizziness, and severe cramping, all of which can be explained with Noakes's "central governor" theory: my body was fighting me to stop moving to prevent, well, death.

In all three cases, I didn't have signs of dehydration or hyponatremia. As such, drinking more or consuming electrolytes had no effect. What *did* help, however, was getting out of the sun and stopping activity. *That* allowed my core temperature to cool.

Some basic experiments seem to support this theory. I did two runs up a mountain, which had several "microclimates" of various combinations of sun exposure and wind. The goal was to try to replicate the feelings of fatigue, dizziness, and cramping without having to run a crazy long distance. I accomplished this by running at a strenuous pace up the mountain. I made sure I was adequately hydrated and electrolytes were supplemented before the run to help rule those out as confounding variables. I carried one water bottle and drank to quench my thirst throughout the run, which equaled about twelve ounces per hour.

The Results

I was able to mimic the exact same feelings I had in the three disastrous runs, though to a lesser degree. The symptoms were worse in sun-exposed areas with no wind, improved in the sun-exposed areas with wind and shaded areas with no wind, and completely disappeared in shaded areas with wind.

I was shocked the results were so clear. Previously, I was at a complete loss as to the cause of the symptoms because I didn't consider body temperature to be a variable. It was never an issue in years of prior running, even when air temps were very high.

As soon as I recognized body temperature was a variable, the correlations became obvious. If sweat isn't cooling me down, performance suffers. A lot.

The Solution

The solutions are obvious: work on methods to stay cool. Here are the steps you can take:

- **Train in heat more often.** Theoretically, this will help make the body's thermoregulation system more efficient. At the very least, it will help train you to recognize the early signs of overheating.
- **In hot, dry weather, go shirtless.** This will maximize evaporative cooling.
- **If there's a lot of sun exposure, wear white cotton shirts.** The white cotton will absorb less heat than skin. The cotton, when saturated with sweat, will allow evaporative

cooling via conduction. I don't think it is as efficient as bare skin, but it is far better than the moisture-wicking materials I've used previously. Also, I've run in cotton in the same hot, dry environments with no issues at all.

- **Use cold water when available.** During a race, I take advantage of cold water (from aid stations or streams) and ice/snow by wrapping it in a bandana and placing it around my neck, dumping it over my head, or some variation of submerging myself. This cools the body via conduction.

- **If all else fails, slow down.** Since movement generates heat, a lack of movement will cool the body quickly. I won't be so stubborn with stopping in the future.

In essence, we have to start treating thermoregulation as a separate variable that's not necessarily controlled by drinking more or popping more salt tabs. That blog post proved to be rather controversial . . . until people actually tried it. If you find yourself having problems in hotter weather, consider clothing choice and the effects of thermoregulation.

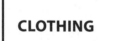

CLOTHING

While I'm a proponent of naked running (give it a shot sometime), society dictates we wear clothing most of the time. I've experimented with all kinds of clothing ranging from simple cotton shorts and T-shirts acquired from Goodwill to the latest scientifically developed technical clothing. I've even tried completely idiotic stuff like skin-tight pleather pants. Even though every shred of common sense may say otherwise, you occasionally find a diamond in the rough. Worth noting: *pleather isn't one of those diamonds.*

Conditions dictate clothing choice. The clothes used for hot, dry weather will obviously be different than overnight runs in freezing, windy conditions. Your own experimentation will help you make the appropriate choices, but here are a few general guidelines:

- **In cold weather, layers are desirable.** The heat generated via muscle contractions should keep you warm. Stopping is troublesome once you get sweaty. As the sweat evaporates, your body cools rapidly. A moisture-wicking underlayer helps draw sweat away from the body, which helps keep you relatively dry. In very cold weather, I like to use a cotton middle layer. This adds warmth without unnecessary bulk. Finally, a wind and/ or waterproof but breathable outer layer will provide a barrier against the elements. Generally speaking, the "technology" of advanced fabrics is a waste of money. Cold weather gear is an exception. The new stuff really is worth the money.

- **In hot weather, less is more.** The human body is especially well-developed for hot weather running as long as sweat is allowed to evaporate from our skin. Many runners like to use moisture-wicking clothing in hot weather, which is a mistake discussed in the previous Thermoregulation section. The more bare skin you can expose, the better. There is an exception to this, however. If you're running in an area with a lot of direct sunlight (like Death Valley), wearing white clothing will reflect more heat than your darker skin.

- **Alternative choices.** Some clothing may seem like a weird option but can work really well. For example, I experimented endlessly with kilts. They allowed me to go commando, which kept my junk cooler and drier and also cut down on salt deposit–induced chafing. Also, I'm a closet exhibitionist.

Wide-brimmed straw gardening hats worked well in hot weather. They're lightweight, sweat-proof, allow sweat on the head to evaporate, reflect heat from above, and shade the upper torso. I also found cotton pajama pants to be ideal nighttime running pants. The thin cotton was breathable but still provided a degree of insulation. They aren't very good if you're running hard, however. You need something more restrictive to hide erections.

Some clothing is worn for support purposes. I was running with two women for a while during a race and the topic drifted to sports bras. One woman asked the other if a sports bra was an absolute requirement. She responded "If guys regularly notice the color of your eyes, you probably don't need one." It seemed like solid advice.

SUNSCREEN

Throughout my formative years, I was taught sunscreen was necessary protection against the evil that is sunlight. Regular exposure to that big ball of fire in the sky would lead to certain death. When I was in college, I would dutifully slather my exposed areas with a liberal handful of SPF 600. Of course, the fact that I attended a college just south of the Arctic Circle (Northern Michigan University on the southern shore of Lake Superior) meant that my "exposed areas" consisted of the skin between my eyes. That trend continued until Shelly and I were expecting our first child. When researching parenting issues, I came across some articles that suggested American children were facing a health crisis due to a lack of vitamin D. Apparently American kids were developing rickets at an unprecedented rate. Why? Parents were coating their children in so much sunscreen their bodies weren't able to produce enough vitamin D (which is manufactured by the body in response to sun exposure). In response, I only used sunscreen if I was going to be exposed for long periods of time.

Years later, I heard of an even more intriguing theory: sun exposure reduced the mortality from internal cancers (cancers other than skin cancer). I first heard of this from Dr. Gordon Ainsleigh, known among ultrarunners as the original runner of the Western States Endurance Run. Gordy published an article in 1993 that has led to more research on the topic (*www.ncbi.nlm. nih.gov/pubmed/8475009*). The article suggests regular, moderate sun exposure has significant health benefits.

After exploring the available research, I changed my sunscreen habits. I have a simple rule: *I only use sunscreen if there's a high probability of burning.*

If I'm running long runs in sunny weather, I use sunscreen. If I'm running in the mountains where the higher altitude results in more intense sun exposure, I wear sunscreen. If I'm running an ultra in sunny weather, I wear sunscreen. Other than those specific situations, I now forgo the sunscreen. It is a philosophy based on the lesser of two evils (skin versus internal cancers), and I try to mitigate the risk by covering up when possible and frequently inspecting my own skin for any abnormalities.

GEAR

Every piece of gear you carry should serve a specific purpose based on the worst case scenario you'll face. If you're running in an urban park with a group of friends, there's no need for survival gear. Leave the fire starter and snakebite kit at home. If you're running on backcountry trails in colder weather, you should carry gear that will allow you to survive in the event something catastrophic occurs.

It is also important to know how to use all of your gear. A GPS watch or emergency beacon is of little use if you don't know how to use it. It's also useful to understand all of the *potential* uses for your gear. For example, a bandana is usually used to shade the head or neck. It can also be used to cool the body when wet, cover the face during a sandstorm or heavy winds, filter sediment from water or extract water from mud, as a tourniquet, shredded and used as a fire starter, cut into lengths and braided into rope, or used to wipe your ass if you have to drop a deuce. All gear has the potential for multiple uses, and knowing those uses will reduce the amount of gear that must be carried into the field.

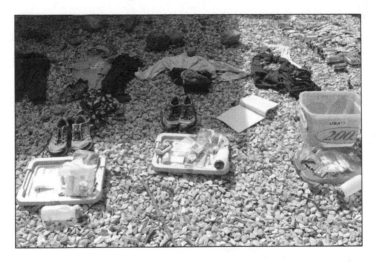

My gear for the Grindstone 100.

TREKKING POLES

Trekking poles are popular among mountain trail runners. They provide extra leverage when ascending and support when descending. They can also be used to help prevent falls.

Personally I hate trekking poles because they're difficult to use in conjunction with handheld water bottles. I also don't like carrying poles on flat sections of the trail. If you do a lot of mountain trail running, borrow a pair and try them on a few runs. You may love them. Or hate them. Or find they're wellsuited for specific conditions.

SHOES

The shoes you choose to wear for trail running should reflect the conditions and terrain you'll encounter. Some conditions may warrant heavy, durable shoes with aggressive tread and a sturdy rock plate (hard piece of plastic embedded in the sole of the shoe to protect the foot from sharp rocks). On nontechnical or even moderately technical trails, road running shoes or even minimalist shoes can be used. With practice, many of those trails could be run barefoot.

So how do you go about choosing shoes? I weigh these variables:

- **Tread:** The tread of the shoe refers to the knobs on the bottom of the sole. This is what grips the terrain. Large, prominent knobs, much like cleats, will be useful in loose dirt, sand, or muddy conditions. Smaller knobs with less space in between are useful for harder surfaces. For bare rock or very hard trails, there's no need for a knobbed tread. The composition of the rubber used for the sole is also significant. Some compounds are "stickier" than others and will grip rocks better than harder compounds. The trade-off is usually durability—softer, stickier compounds wear faster than the harder compounds.

- **Sole protection:** The stack height, or thickness of the sole, will determine how much protection the shoe provides. A thicker sole will provide more protection. As mentioned above, the presence of a rock plate also adds protection. The more technical the trail, the more protection is needed and the thicker the sole must be. The trade-off is ground feel and proprioception. "Ground feel" is the ability to feel the terrain under foot. Many people prefer as minimal a shoe as possible because it helps traverse difficult terrain. Proprioception is our awareness of body position. A thinner sole allows for better proprioception, which helps prevent injuries like sprained ankles.

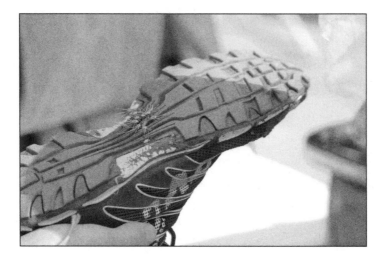

- **Cushioning:** Cushioning refers to the "give" of the shoe under foot. A shoe with more cushioning has more of a marshmallow feel, whereas a shoe with less cushioning will feel harder. Cushioning can provide additional comfort when running longer distances. The tradeoff is efficiency—the more cushioning under foot, the less "springiness" the legs have. That loss of springiness may have a negative impact on efficiency.

- **Heel drop:** Heel drop refers to the difference in stack height as measured in the center of the heel and the center of the area under the ball of the foot. The drop is usually measured in millimeters expressed as "eight-millimeter drop." The vast majority of shoes either have a "zero-drop" heel where the measurements are the same, or have a slightly raised heel. Raising the heel will affect posture, which may cause unnecessary stresses on the lower back and knees. Because of this, I prefer shoes with a four-millimeter drop or less. Shoes that have a greater drop alter your posture just like a stripper wearing four-inch stilettos. They cause your chest and ass to stick out. Cool effect for the stage . . . not so much out on the trails.

- **Upper:** The upper is the top part of the shoe that encases the foot. Uppers are chosen based on comfort and conditions. Some shoes have a softer, more flexible upper. This adds to comfort but may cause the shoe to move around on the foot. This is especially problematic when running downhill. Stiffer uppers help secure the shoe to the foot, but may not be as comfortable. Many uppers are now being designed with little or no internal seams so they can be worn without socks. Some uppers are made to resist water for use in rainy weather or trails with many water crossings. Others are designed with insulation for cold weather running. Choose the shoe that appropriately matches the conditions.

- **Ventilation:** Ventilation refers to the breathability of the shoe, or the ability for air circulation. Greater ventilation keeps your feet cool and dry. It also allows debris like dust and sand to enter the shoe.

- **Shape of last:** The "last" is the device used to mold the shoe during the manufacturing process. Different manufacturers use different lasts, and many manufacturers use multiple lasts. Last shape tends to be a matter of personal preference. I prefer an "anatomical last" that conforms to the shape of the human foot. This reduces the rubbing between my foot and the inside of the shoe, which allows me to run sockless without blistering. My best advice: try several brands and models of shoes until you find a last you prefer.

ILLUMINATION

If you plan to do any nighttime trail running, illumination of some sort is pretty much a necessity. Some trails can be safely navigated by street lighting (like urban parks) or moonlight during a full moon, but most require a light. The options are handheld flashlights or headlamps. If you're a hipster, you could probably get away with a flaming torch.

Many people prefer headlamps. I don't like headlamps because the light is too close to one's eyes. The shadows cast by the light make it almost impossible to see, which makes it difficult to determine the exact height of debris on the trail. A handheld carried at about waist level casts shadows on a different plane, which makes obstacle discrimination far easier.

My current preference is the Fenix brand of handhelds. They make several models that use standard AA batteries (easy to find), last through the night, are extremely durable, and are ridiculously bright. As mentioned earlier, one can also be used as a kubotan in an emergency. My preferred model throws 190 lumens (the measure of the light produced by any given source), which more or less turns the night to day. The light is so bright it can even turn some fabrics transparent . . . or so I'm told. This is the same flashlight I mention in the "Personal Protection" section, so it can double as a weapon. If you need other options, ask a spelunker.

In the event you're ever stranded on the trail in darkness and have no light, you can easily enhance your night vision. I learned this trick from a grizzled old raccoon hunter in northern Michigan. First, don't move during civil twilight, or the point where all light disappears from the sky. It takes about thirty minutes for your eyes to fully adjust to the darkness. When your eyes adjust to the darkness, look to the *side* of an object you're looking at. Our eyes "see" using cells called rods and cones. Rods are primarily responsible for low light vision and have a higher concentration in the parts of our eyes that register peripheral vision. At night, you can't see an object quite as well if you look directly at it. It's bizarre to be able to see something better by not looking directly at it. In fact, it usually takes a little bit of time to suppress the urge to stare at whatever you're trying to see.

BEARDS

Trail and ultrarunning results in some strange stylistic fads. I like to think I've always been at the cutting edge of ultrarunning hipsterdom with styles like kilts, pajama pants, and cotton in lieu of moisture-wicking shirts. I was a late-adopter for one particular fad, however: beards.

At the time of writing (late 2013), beards are all the rage in the trail running scene. Some folks have been rocking the full beard for decades (Gordy Ainsleigh), while others have only been doing it for a number of years (Tony Krupicka). Personally, I've always enjoyed facial hair because a) I'm lazy, and b) the shit grows like weeds. I can grow a full beard in about two weeks. If I went with the clean-shaven look, the cost of razors would probably have used up my entire ultrarunning budget.

There are pros and cons to the bearded look. Let's explore the negatives first.

- It can scare little kids. And their overprotective parents.
- Some women (or men) do not like the look or feel.
- Sometimes food gets stuck in the nest.
- It *can* be hot in the summer.
- Some employers frown upon facial hair.

Of course, all of these "cons" could really be "pros" in disguise. Little kids are annoying and keeping them away isn't a bad thing. Women (or men) who don't like beards probably wouldn't be cool with trail running and ultramarathons, so it can be a nice "mate-selection" filter. Food getting stuck? Can you say "between-meal snack?" Summer heat? Just douse the beard with water to create a face-cooling heat exchanger. Employers who frown upon facial hair? That's basically the same as mate selection. Do you really want to work for someone who doesn't appreciate facial hair?

So what about the pros?

- Manliness factor
- Protection from the elements: wind, cold, and snow
- Facial camouflage to hide a weak chin
- Saves time and money due to the absence of shaving
- French tickler

To me, the choice seems obvious. If you *can* grow a beard, you *need* to grow a beard.

CARRYING WATER

Most people use one of three options for carrying water or sports drinks. They use handheld water bottles, hydration packs that are affixed to the back, or complicated fanny packs that carry water bottles. Each one has pros and cons.

- **Handhelds**: Handhelds have three major advantages. Having your drink in your hands helps you remember to drink regularly, offers some hand protection should you fall, and are easy to fill at aid stations. The downside to handhelds is weight. It can be difficult to carry a twenty- to twenty-four ounce water bottle all day. Also, I've had some problems with the strap on the water bottle chafing my knuckles.

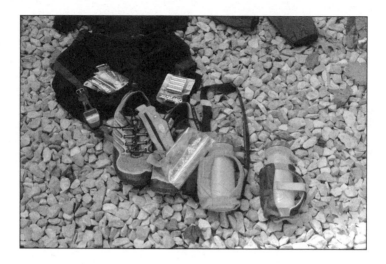

- **Hydration packs**: Hydration packs hold far more of your favorite beverage than handhelds, and the weight is equally distributed on your back. The backpacks can bounce around if your running form is too "bouncy" (see the section on good form). Hydration packs are also a pain in the ass to fill at aid stations, though you have to fill them less often.
- **Fanny packs**: In my opinion, these are the worst of both worlds. The water bottles are held around your butt, which requires reaching back to grab. Since the bottles are out of sight, there's no reminder to drink. Finally, the pack itself may cause chafing due to bouncing.

It is possible to run without anything and just rely on the aid stations. I wouldn't advise this if you are a new ultrarunner, especially if it is hot or the aid stations are farther than five miles apart.

KNOWING WHERE TO FIND WATER

When it comes to training, hydration can be a bitch. Once the long runs surpass your ability to physically carry enough water (or other drink), your options are limited. You can:

- Stash drinks along the planned route in some sort of jug or container (though they may get stolen . . . which has happened on more than one occasion. Seriously, who steals a jug of water?) A related option is to plan a loop route that will take you back to your vehicle.
- Bring money or a credit card if there will be stores along the way.
- Plan a route that utilizes public drinking fountains.
- Bogart water from your running partners, or take it by force if they refuse to comply.

Personally, I prefer the drinking fountains. If you live in a semi-inhabited area, this is a good option. If you live in the sticks or will be training in desolate mountains, it may be impossible. If you do train in a populated area, drinking fountains can usually be found at:

- Public parks and playgrounds
- Sport fields
- Public restrooms
- Schools
- Trailheads
- Campgrounds
- Large grocery, department, or other such stores
- Malls

WATER FROM NATURAL SOURCES

You're out on a long run and your bottle goes dry. You start experiencing the early signs of dehydration. You are nowhere near a drinking fountain or a store. What do you do?

I've run into this scenario many times over the years . . . and I always choose the same course of action: I scavenge for water anywhere I can. That has included drinking from streams, lakes, or a water hose in some random person's yard, or making a funnel out of a leaf during a rainstorm.

There's always an inherent danger in drinking water from questionable sources. The water may contain organisms that can make you sick, like giardia or dysentery. The water could also be contaminated with poisons that could kill you. It's always a gamble.

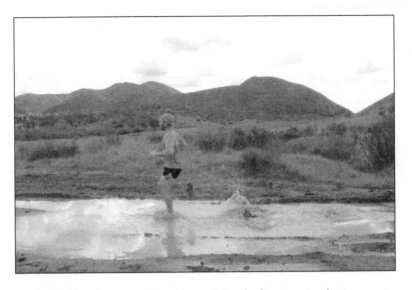

In an emergency situation, I look for water that contains some form of life. If a water source does not have any signs of life (fish, plants, etc.), odds are pretty good that it's undrinkable due to some horrific contamination. Next, I make a filter out of a bandana and a water bottle by placing the bandana over the mouth of the bottle and attaching it with rubber bands (I keep a few rubber bands wrapped around all my water bottles). When the bottle is submerged, the bandana acts as a filter. It's not nearly as effective as boiling water, using a commercial filter, or chemically purifying the water, but rarely do I, if ever, have the tools required for elaborate purification. The homemade filter will likely trap most of the harmful stuff and is better than drinking straight from the questionable source.

If you have access to a piece of plastic or a space blanket and a container of some sort, you can make a solar still. A water bottle works well. The setup will use evaporation to purify water over the course of several hours. Here's how to construct the still:

1. Dig a hole eighteen inches deep by twenty-four inches wide in a sunny area.
2. Line the hole with one piece of plastic.
3. Place a small rock or mound of dirt in the middle of the plastic.
4. Place your container on the mound.
5. Dump contaminated water, urine, or green plants in the hole.
6. Cover the entire hole with another piece of plastic and secure it in place by placing rocks or dirt around the edge. The better the coverage, the better the still will work.
7. Place a small pebble on top of the cover sheet directly above the mouth of the container.

How it works: The still works when the sun heats the contaminated water, urine, or plants, which evaporates the water. The evaporated water collects on the bottom of the cover sheet. The pebble in the middle causes the water to run down the sheet and drip in the bottle. If you don't have enough plastic or you have no water or plants to place in the hole, skip the liner from step two. The still will draw moisture from the ground.

If you're near a water source like a river, stream, or a beach and you can build a fire, the process can be expedited. Dig a hole near the water source deep enough so the bottom fills with water. Place a container in the center, and then partially cover the hole with the plastic. Build a fire a few feet from the hole. Place a few rocks in the fire. After a few minutes, use a stick to move the hot rocks into the water hole, then immediately cover the hole with the plastic and drop a pebble above the mouth of the container. After a few minutes, place the rocks back in the fire and repeat.

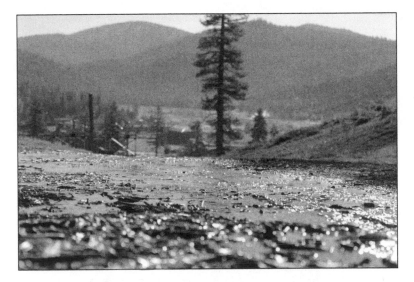

Water can also be extracted from mud with the use of a sock, bandana, shirt, or other fabric. Wrap a softball-size clump of mud in the fabric (or plop it in the sock). Squeeze the fabric over a container. The fabric will effectively hold most of the dirt behind. The water will still have to be purified, however.

To cool the water (or any other liquid), you can once again utilize fabric. Socks work best. Drop the sealed container of water (or beer cans . . . whatever) in the sock. Saturate the sock with water. It doesn't have to be purified water. Hang the sock in a shady area exposed to wind. The blowing aids the evaporation of the water, which cools the liquid in the container. I have Jeremiah Cataldo to thank for that tip.

What if there aren't obvious water sources? Remember water always flows downhill. Birds also tend to congregate near water at dawn and dusk. Look for them circling in the sky. Here are some location-specific places that can be used as, or may lead to, sources of water:

- **Cold environments** - snow and ice
- **Desert** - trails, animal droppings, birds, palm trees, base of hills, or mountains
- **Forest** - animal trails (get wider and deeper toward water source, downhill), birds, insects, and density and "greenness" of plants; if spring bed is dry, dig
- **Mountains** - valleys and crevices in rock (formed by flowing water)
- **Plains** - look for taller vegetation like small trees growing in groups (pond) or a line (stream)

RUNNING WITH KIDS

Running Partners

I'll be completely honest, I have no idea why people would have a desire to run with their children. Getting an hour or so of quiet solitude away from their screaming neediness is the whole reason I continued ultrarunning after our daughter was born. I love my kids, but I also love getting away from them. Shelly and I also spent two years homeschooling them, so that 24/7 exposure gave us more than enough "family time." Running will tire kids out, though. Sleepy kids usually equals happy parents. Running is also great exercise, which is becoming increasingly important in our digital age. If you want to include your children in your trail running adventure, the main consideration is their limitations.

Consider the kid. If this is their first trail run, go slow and keep the distance at a minimum. A short out-and-back route can be good, but a looped course that takes you back to the starting point would be better. Go slow and accommodate for their physical limitations. I would advise against dangerous trail runs that could result in getting lost. Kids make a survival situation more difficult.

Of course, this assumes you're relatively experienced and your child isn't necessarily fit. In the likely (here in America anyway) scenario where you've been a long-term couch potato and your kid is relatively fit, they'll probably run circles around you. The combination of a hyper kid and air-gulping exhaustion can ruin the trail running experience. If that's the case, I'd recommend doing a warmup activity to wear the kids out before hitting the trail. If there's a sizable parking lot, have the kids run a few laps around it. If the terrain has hills, offer to time them as they run to the top. Whatever their times happen to be, tell them you've done it ten seconds faster. Have them repeat the climb until they're sufficiently exhausted.

RUNNING WITH DOGS

As I mentioned earlier, dogs can make ideal training partners. If you're in the market for a dog and your primary goal is to find a running partner, look for a breed that is adept at running. Sled dog breeds, sporting and hunting breeds, and herding dogs all make decent running partners. Chihuahuas and Shih Tzus . . . not so much.

Dogs have issues with thermoregulation. They cannot run in hot weather like humans. Humans can cool down while moving due to our sweating mechanism; dogs will pant to cool down and will need to stop moving if they overheat. If your dog wants to stop and lie down, it's too hot. Don't continue forcing it to run. If you live in a warm or hot climate, you will probably have to run early in the morning, late in the evening, or at night.

Dogs need to work up to longer distances, just like we do. If their first run is a twenty-miler, odds are good they'll get hurt. Get a good leash, and avoid retractable leashes. Take time training the dog. Before taking your dog out on the trails, it should be able to reliably come when called, sit, stay, and be able to run at your side without excessive pulling.

ENCOUNTERING OTHER DOGS ON THE TRAIL

Sometimes when running you'll encounter strays or other people's dogs. It would be great to automatically assume every dog has a "Lassie-esque" temperament. Sadly, that's not the case. All dogs share a great deal of genetic material with their wolf cousins. As such, the "kill" instinct is still present. We often make the mistake of assuming dogs act like humans and place ourselves in really bad situations. Dogs aren't people; don't make the mistake of anthropomorphizing them.

If you encounter any dog, the first step is to assess its behavior. Is it a potential threat or is it friendly? It's safe to assume *all* dogs can be a danger, but some dogs will be more dangerous than others—different dogs have different aggressive signals. Some will lower their heads, lower their tails, make eye contact, bare their teeth, and approach you on a direct line. Others may raise their heads, ears, and tails high to appear taller. The one common denominator: relaxation. An aggressive dog will almost always show a fight or flight response—they look tense.

On the other hand, a friendly dog will look relaxed, almost like a googly-eyed drunk Muppet. This can sometimes be

113

deceiving unless you've spent a lot of time around different dogs. Furthermore, even a friendly dog can be overexcited and bite.

I use caution with all dogs due to this ambiguity. If I see a dog on the trail, I step off to the side, avoid direct eye contact, and wait for it to pass. If the dog seems really aggressive, I may *slowly* back away. The key is to avoid triggering the dog's predator response or appearing to be a threat.

If the dog is aggressive and isn't leaving or appears to be preparing to attack, it's decision time. Our first human instinct is to run. If you can flee to a safe place (car, tree, house, Waffle House, etc.) before the dog can reach you, running isn't such a bad choice. The dog *will* be chasing you, and it will be biting you to drag you to the ground.

If you can't escape quickly, the other option is to fight. Sometimes a fight can be avoided by intimidating the dog by loudly and aggressively screaming. Some dogs will back down in the face of bat-shit crazy. If it's a guard dog or a stereotypically aggressive breed like pit bulls, German shepherds, rottweilers, etc., using this tactic may anger them. Let's assume your intimidation ploy didn't work.

In the best-case scenario, you came prepared and can use a weapon (gun, pepper spray, knife, stun gun, drum stick . . . whatever) to protect yourself. If there's a stick or rock nearby, that can be used, too. An attacking dog will be fast, so you won't have much time to react. Depending on the weapon, it may be more effective to wait for the dog to reach you. Stay on your feet. Keep something between your body and the dog. Your nondominant forearm will work. When the dog clamps on, use the weapon.

If you're unarmed, assume you're going to get bitten. A lot. Use the same tactic. Stay on your feet and get something between you and the dog. If you're using your forearm, don't pull it away when the dog bites. This natural reaction will cause more damage. Instead, try to thrust your hand down the dog's throat. If that's not possible, aggressively gouge the dog's eye with your other thumb. By "aggressively" I mean "try to remove the eye from the socket." If the dog is still biting, go for the other eye. If that doesn't work, the next best option is to attempt to choke the dog out by cutting off the blood supply to its brain by applying pressure to both carotid arteries toward the front of the dog's neck. If the blood supply is completely cut off, the dog will lose consciousness in less than ten seconds. In 2009, a nine-year-old boy, Drew Heredia, saved a twelve-year-old girl's life by applying a rear naked choke to an attacking pit bull. Need a better reason to add MMA or jujitsu to your cross-training routine?

If you happen to be attacked by a pack of dogs and you're unarmed . . . well, hopefully you've been serious about finishing that bucket list.

Seriously though, a pack makes defense infinitely more difficult. It's not like a 1970s kung fu movie where one attacks while the others patiently wait their turn. They all attack at the same time; that's part of the reason they hunt in packs. Watch this video, then imagine you're the bison: *www.youtube.com/watch?v=CT_3QiWQh8M.*

If you are attacked by a pack, don't have weapons, and cannot quickly escape to a secure area, try the intimidation trick. If that fails, identifying the alpha, or the pack leader; taking them out may cause the others to leave. Of course, modern canine experts have cast doubt on the idea that alphas even exist. The lesson: it's not a bad idea to carry a weapon of some sort.

RUNNING WITH CATS

When Shelly and I were traveling around the United States in our RV, we encountered some weird folks. Some were even weirder than us, which is quite an accomplishment. One of the most bizarre things we saw were cats being walked on leashes. Most of these people were older retirees. This makes sense because the transient owners are worried about the welfare of their cats. They could get lost, run over if they wander to adjacent highways, attacked by dogs, etc. We currently own a cat and tried walking him on a leash. It went over about as well as the day the kids tried dragging him in a campground hot tub.

One cat/leash incident stands out. We were camping in Virginia as I was preparing for the Grindstone hundred-miler. I was doing a morning cross-training workout on the shore of the small lake owned by the campground. Each morning, I saw a younger (early thirties) dude dressed in running gear while walking through the campground into the nearby forest with his leashed cat in tow. After a few days my curiosity got the better of me. I approached him and asked him how he trained his cat to walk on the leash, using the cover story of my desire to walk our own cat. According to his story, the cat always seemed to enjoy the leashed walks, which he had done since it was a kitten. Much to my surprise, he also explained the cat wasn't as fond of running on a leash. When he disappeared into the forest, he actually did some trail running with the cat. I was flabbergasted.

The secret to his feline running partner success: *Let the cat lead the way.* This advice shouldn't come as a surprise to cat owners. Cats have the rebelliousness of teenagers and the apathy of serial killers. If you have a cat and want to convert it to a running partner, it's possible. It's also possible to become a professional rattlesnake masseuse.

RUNNER PERSONALITIES

As runners, most of us fit in one of two categories: we strive to improve our abilities, or we accept our abilities and focus on the enjoyment of running. The vast majority of runners will be some combination of these two extremes, but will be a little closer to one side or the other.

Both approaches have distinct advantages and disadvantages. If you strive to improve your abilities, you'll actually improve your running skills. You'll be able to run longer, faster, or both. You'll likely identify weaknesses in your running abilities and take steps to improve. There are downsides, too. You may never feel quite satisfied. You could have always run a little faster or longer, or there will always be someone that does a little better.

If you're not chasing authentic goals (goals you set as opposed to goals that are set for you by others), you may end up with a hollow sense of accomplishment. Lastly, you may look down on other runners who don't share the desire to constantly improve.

The "running for enjoyment" personality has advantages, too. You're likely going to play to your strengths. If you're a road runner, you'll stick to roads. You're also more likely to be happy with your current situation. You don't need to accomplish anything to feel good about yourself. Lastly, you'll be more likely to accept others for the runners they are without judging their abilities or performances. There are downsides to this mind-set, too. You may feel like you're not really accomplishing anything. You may feel your approach is just an excuse to be a lazy ass. You may shun others because they try to be competitive or improve regularly. Finally, you may not be a good advocate for the sport.

As you can probably guess, extremes of either are not good. Striking a happy balance is probably the ideal.

TRAINING RUN CONVERSATIONS

Now that you have a training partner, you may need some help with conversation topics. Well, if you have social skills like me, you could use some help. The rest of you socially competent folks are fine; go ahead and skip this section.

Those long runs can last forever, so these should help fill the awkward lulls. I'm dividing the topics based on familiarity with the training partner.

Partner you just met:

- Weather
- Movies you've recently watched
- Running history, how and why you started
- Profession
- Kids (if you have them . . . otherwise pets are acceptable)

Someone you've known for a few weeks:

- Educational history
- Family history
- Food preferences/diet
- Observations about other runners you see on the trail, but stay positive
- Favorite childhood cartoons and/or toys

Someone you've been running with for months:

- Political views
- Religious views
- Philosophy of life
- Dreams and aspirations
- Whether you sleep in the nude or prefer pajamas
- Annoying coworkers

Someone you've been running with for at least a year:

- Details of the poop you just took in the woods (color, consistency, etc.)
- How different sports bras and/or shorts keep your breasts and/or genitals from bouncing

- Your real dreams and aspirations that you were too embarrassed to admit earlier
- Your top five erogenous zones
- Best place to dispose of the bodies of those annoying coworkers
- That trip to Cancun, the video on the Internet, and your resulting illegitimate child

HOW TO GET RID OF THAT ANNOYING TRAINING PARTNER

I've been lucky—all of my training partners have been great. However, I do occasionally get questions about annoying training partners. Specifically, how you gracefully get rid of them. Here are some approaches:

Method One: Be direct. Simply tell them "I don't want to run with you anymore. You annoy the shit out of me." If you want to make it more dramatic, add something like, "Remember on our last run when you talked nonstop for six hours about how barefoot running changed your life? I spent the entire time contemplating the pros and cons of murder versus suicide." This is probably the healthiest approach and the only one I'd recommend. Maybe skip that last part.

Method Two: Be passive aggressive. This rarely works and is totally unhealthy, but some people find it fun. Or it's a manifestation of a fucked-up childhood. Start by showing up fifteen minutes late to every run. Next, escalate it by having them run first on trails through wooded areas so they hit all the spider webs spanning across the trail. When running side by side, most of us like to run on one side or the other. Figure out their preference then always run on the *opposite* side.

If they duck off the trail to relieve themselves, tell them you'll be the lookout. Look the other way when another runner approaches so they're caught in a compromising position. Finally, invite them to a Mexican restaurant the night before a long run. Insist on ordering a bean-heavy dish. The next day, mix up the antidiarrhea medication with a laxative, tell them you'll bring the toilet paper on the run, and then conveniently forget it at home.

Method Three: Out-annoy them. The idea is to escalate every annoying thing they say. For example, if they say "I'm a Republican and I believe we should have guns!" You respond with "Damn right we should have guns! How else are we going to launch the revolution? In fact, we're having a meeting tomorrow night, and you're just the kind of person we're looking for! By the way, what's your blood type?" If you fancy yourself as a comedian, try offensive humor. If they're hard-core Christians, try "Jesus walks into Courtyard by Marriot, throws three nails down on the counter, and asks 'Can you put me up for the night?'"

If none of these methods are effective, you can always plant a bag of weed in their hydration pack and report them to the cops.

BURNING RIVER PART I

After my broken-toe fifty-miler, I had plenty of downtime to consider my next goal. I really wanted to run a hundred-miler, even though my fifty didn't go as well as planned. I scoured the race calendars and found a good race relatively close to home: the Burning River 100 in Ohio. The race was a point-to-point race that started in a suburb of Cleveland and ran south near the Cuyahoga River. According to reports the course would be barefoot friendly, support was excellent, and the scenery was pleasant.

I knew I needed a different training routine; my previous one just didn't cut it. I searched around for a while and came to the conclusion that I needed to add less "bodybuilding" weight training, more high rep/low weight training, and speedwork. While looking for plans, I came across a few YouTube videos for "Gym Jones," a private gym in Utah. They were doing some crazy timed circuit training workouts. Having studied physical education in college, I was familiar with the principles of the workouts, but hadn't considered the application to running really long, slow distances.

I did a little more research and came across a crude website known as "Crossfit" and a variation known as "Crossfit Endurance." This is the same plan I mentioned in the cross-training section earlier. I read some of their links to published research and decided this was the plan for me. Yes, I'm playing the exercise hipster card. I was doing Crossfit before CF "boxes" became the Starbucks of gyms where they can be now found on any street corner.

The Crossfit workouts used a lot of high-intensity interval training coupled with some Olympic and power lifting barbell lifts. The Crossfit Endurance workouts involved a lot of speed-work and other higher intensity running workouts. The one thing that was noticeably absent: the long run. The logic made sense. The shorter, faster runs coupled with the weight training prepared the body without the negative impact of the long, slow runs (increased injuries, muscle atrophy, etc.).

The lack of long runs freed up quite a bit of time, which I used to obsessively plan every detail for the race. I probably made three hundred spreadsheets that winter and spring. I made elaborate pace charts using math skills I didn't know I had. I read every race report for the race. I memorized the elevation chart and aid stations. I watched video of most of the course.

Given Burning River was so much longer than my previous fifty-milers, I decided to enlist the help of a crew and pacers. I didn't know too many runners at the time, so I had two non-ultrarunner friends, Jason Saint Amour and Rich Elliott, help me out. Since we didn't have a lot of time to collaborate, I made a complex set of directions to sort out all of the crap I was planning on taking. I knew all of the possible pitfalls of running a hundred-miler based on my readings and I thought I would be ready. I made contingency plans, and contingency plans for the contingency plans.

When the race rolled around, I was ready. We loaded Rich's van with the gear and made the drive from Grand Rapids to Cleveland. On the way, we skipped talk of race logistics in favor of our favorite nude scenes from movies and sub-par beer we drank in college. I may have mentioned something about pace charts and drop bags once or twice. I was getting nervous but had confidence in my plan.

The next morning, I was following my to-do prerace list. I showered, lubed the areas that would chafe, and got dressed. As I was filling my water bottle, I noticed my watch was missing. I need it to track my pace from one aid station to the next. In a panic, I gathered up our gear and checked out of the hotel so we would have time to find an open store that sold watches.

There's a funny thing about suburban Cleveland: everything is closed on Saturday mornings. Grocery stores, pharmacies, department stores . . . even gas stations were closed. We were running low on time so I had Rich and Jason drop me off at the start line. After the race started, they'd continue searching for a watch.

Standing at the start line, barefoot, in the dark was a surreal experience. I knew I was about to embark on the most difficult journey of my life, but I was strangely calm. The previous nervousness seemed to disappear. Maybe it was the jovial, joking attitude of the other runners; maybe it was the cool, wet grass under my feet. Regardless, I was in a good place.

The race start, like most ultras, didn't involve too much fanfare. The entire first eighteen miles or so were on asphalt and were rather easy. I went out a little too fast but was able to reign myself in after my crew scored a watch. After about twenty-five miles, I started to develop some crazy-annoying sensitivity on the soles of my feet. It became apparent I wouldn't be able to run barefoot too much longer. At the next aid station, I slipped into my trusty Vibram Five Fingers KSOs. They felt unusually tight, but I ignored it. That turned out to be a major mistake. I didn't consider my feet would swell, and my KSOs were far too small to accommodate my expanding feet. I spent the next twenty-five miles fighting off blistering and gradually blackening toenails.

When I rolled into the aid station around mile forty-five, I was feeling unusually good. I was in far better condition at that point than my two previous ultras. I was mentally singing the praises of my Crossfit and Crossfit Endurance training regimen. My crew had developed a fast, efficient aid station routine, I was right around my desired pace, and my feet were the only real problem. This ultrarunning thing was getting pretty easy!

My crew couldn't meet me at that aid station due to access issues, so I was on my own to care for my needs. I chatted with the volunteers, applied some more lube, and filled my water bottle. I wasn't particularly hungry at the moment and nothing sounded good, so I skipped food. "I'll just eat at the next aid station," I reasoned.

Heh. I wouldn't eat another bite for the rest of the race.

Mile fifty was tough. Mile fifty-five was really tough. The pain in my feet was intensifying. My arms and legs started stiffening up; I was chafing. Sunset was fast approaching as I met my crew at the "Boston Store" aid station immediately before a short loop around a dam. I was feeling down but my crew managed to cheer me up. They gave me my flashlight and a piece of pizza and kicked me out of the aid station. As I started down the trail, I took a bite of the pizza. I almost vomited. I tossed it in the bushes.

The next five miles would prove to be the worst experience I've ever had as a runner. As the light disappeared, I experienced what could only be described as extreme physical fatigue coupled with severe depression. The depth of the emotional despair scared me to the point where I had a minor panic attack. I collapsed under a tree, shut off my light, and curled up in the fetal position. I considered my options. I desperately wanted to stop but knew I had several miles to go. I couldn't create a logical argument to pull myself off the ground, so I continued to lie there. I'm not sure what eventually compelled me to get up, but I did. I started a ridiculously slow zombie shuffle along the trail. I came to a small, steep ravine and peered over the edge. About ten feet below were several large, jagged boulders. I came stupidly close to jumping down the ravine knowing I'd hurt myself enough to get out of the race. The only thing that stopped me was the concern that I was now the last runner on the course. It would probably take the rescue crew a long time to find me. I continued shuffling on.

My limping shuffle eventually led me back to the Boston Store aid station. I was unbelievably relieved to finally end the damn race. That is, until I talked to Rich. First, this was the point where I could get a pacer and Rich was scheduled to take the next section. Second, I had told them not to let me drop out under any circumstance. I thought I was too close to the cutoff time, but Rich had persuaded the aid station captain to let me continue. Despite my objections, Rich dragged me back out on the trail.

It was a decision he probably regretted almost immediately. I couldn't go faster than a *very* slow shuffle. I was cold, sleepy, and in incredible pain. I was alternating between hallucinating and blacking out. I couldn't walk in a straight line. I tried convincing Rich to turn around, but he was far too much of an optimist. Oh, I should mention that Rich once ran a marathon with no training. That's not "he ran a marathon without marathon-specific training"; he didn't run *at all*. He ran exactly twenty-six point two miles that year . . . all of it came from the one race.

At some point, Rich gave me a bag of chocolate-coated coffee beans I had prepared a week earlier. In my exercise-induced stupor, I ate the entire bag. There were approximately 110 beans in the bag, each bean containing about seven milligrams of caffeine. I had ingested the equivalent of seven cups of coffee *at one time*. Within fifteen minutes my heart was racing uncontrollably; I was sweating profusely and started shaking. The symptoms were bad enough, but were infinitely worse coupled with all the other problems I had experienced.

It took us somewhere around three hours to "run" about five miles. By the time we reached the next aid station, I was way past the cutoff. The aid station captain officially ended my race. I was relieved but still fighting an unbelievable low. Jason helped me to the van and I washed off as well as I could given my limited mobility. I changed into my pajama pants and hoodie. Rich was still pumped to run, so we drove to the next aid station where he volunteered to pace a runner that didn't have a crew or pacer. I curled up in a ball and fell asleep immediately.

Burning River was my first DNF and it hurt. I had fancied myself as a pretty good runner; reality is a harsh mistress, however. The failure led me to reassess my training (again). It forced me to accept that I couldn't just replicate a prepackaged plan and expect success. I would have to find my own answers. This was the point where I really embraced the idea of self-experimentation. I was going to solve this hundred-mile riddle, damn it!

SECTION 4:
SAFETY AND SURVIVAL

PREPARING FOR TROUBLE

What happens if you get lost? Or hurt? For anyone venturing into the wilderness, this is a real possibility. Preparing for trouble can help keep you safe. The more remote the area, the more important good preparation becomes. Interestingly, I've found this to be more of a male issue than a female issue. It's just like driving a car. If a woman doesn't know where she is or where she's going, she'll stop and ask for directions. Men? We adopt a different strategy. We convince ourselves we know what the hell we're doing, confidently head in a random direction, and end up in an even worse predicament. Gender effects aside, here are some helpful tips.

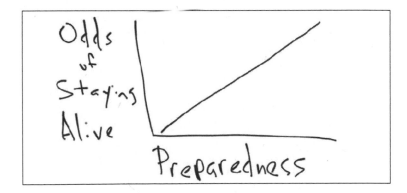

Before You Leave for Your Run

Always tell someone where you are going, when you plan on returning, and who to contact should you fail to return. Exact information could include the trailhead where you will start, the number of people in your running group, gear you are bringing (food, water, fire-starting equipment, clothing, shelter, etc.), your experience level, maps and compass, and your planned route. All of this information can be used by search and rescue to help plan a search effort.

Give the person an exact time you plan on returning, but give yourself some wiggle room in case you're delayed. Instruct him or her to attempt to call you first in case you forget to call him or her. If him or her doesn't get a response, give him or her an emergency contact number based on the area you're running. He or she will forward all your information to the authorities, who will forward it to the search and rescue agency.

In the event this isn't possible, you can leave a note with the same information in your car at the trailhead. If you don't return, search and rescue will locate and search your car. I've never been a fan of this because I don't want to advertise my whereabouts and return time to prospective thieves. If you do this, leave the note folded on the dashboard. If the trailhead has a register, fill it out. Search and rescue will also use this to locate you. Don't pull an Aron Ralston.

If You Do Get Lost or Hurt

Knowing how search and rescue operates is useful to maximize their efforts to find you. First, stabilize any injuries and move to a safe place. For example, if you're bleeding, stop it. If you're on top of a summit during a thunderstorm, move to lower ground. If you're in a floodplain during a rain storm, move to higher ground.

Second, assess the situation. If there's a very good chance of finding your way out of trouble in a timely manner, a storm is closing in and you don't have a means of building a shelter, or you didn't tell anyone where you're running, try navigating out.

If not, stay put. If people are searching for you, moving makes it much more difficult to locate you.

This is the process SAR usually uses to locate lost runners. Search and rescue efforts usually start with teams checking obvious locations in the event you're not really lost, like your tent, car, or home. This is done in the event you didn't have a means (or forgot) to contact the person who reported you missing.

The SAR team begins the actual search by determining your last-known location. They calculate the time that has elapsed since you were last seen and how fast you were likely traveling. Using this data, they can determine the size of the search area.

Before beginning the actual search, the SAR team will post people on roads, trails, and streams or rivers around the boundary of the search area. This serves two purposes: if you're moving, there's a chance you will run into one of the SAR team members; it also helps assure the search area doesn't enlarge over time since it will be unlikely you'll pass by one of the containment team members. This is the reason staying in one place is important— moving out of this search zone will *dramatically* increase the time it takes to find you, since the initial search zone will be thoroughly searched first.

The search team will then dispatch small teams to quickly search the zone. They will check any place people may go when lost or injured such as shelters or caves, or check obviously dangerous places like cliffs. The goal of this stage is to end the search quickly, so the searchers aren't especially thorough.

Shortly after, SAR may dispatch helicopters or airplanes to search from the air. They will look for signs like fires, shelters, or signals and notes left on the ground. They may or may not use heat-detecting technology.

SAR may also use signaling methods like whistles, car horns, or yelling. If you hear any of these, attempt to respond. If possible, head toward the signals. It's a good idea to mark your path in some way. This allows you to return to your shelter if needed and creates a series of clues if SAR stumbles upon your path.

If the initial search is unsuccessful, the SAR team may expand the search zone or, more likely, use a grid search of the area. The team will section off the area, then have searchers thoroughly search each section of the grid for any clue they can find. This is a very slow, manpower-intensive process usually reserved for times when looking for an incapacitated person or a body.

You can greatly increase your chances of being found by following a few guidelines that will assist SAR.

Step 1: Get safe. If you're in a dangerous place (possible rock slides, avalanche zone, ridge or summit during a thunderstorm, a flood plane, etc.), move to a safe location. If you're injured, administer appropriate first aid.

Step 2: Protect yourself from the elements. The greatest danger in a survival situation is exposure. Heat or cold can kill a human surprisingly fast. If you are close to a known shelter, take refuge there. SAR will likely search those first, so it increases your odds of being found. If not, use whatever you have at your disposal to build a makeshift shelter. If you are prepared, you should have an emergency blanket and some cord. This can be combined with trees, sticks, or other natural elements to build a simple lean-to shelter.

Shelter placement is a trade-off between visibility and protection. If you built the shelter in an open area, it is more likely to be seen from above. However, it also exposes you to the elements. It's probably a better idea to build the shelter near a bare hilltop or clearing, then construct signaling devices in the open areas.

This step should also include building a fire if the weather is colder. A small fire built near the open side of a lean-to with a reflector on the opposite side will provide plenty of warmth.

Step 3: Build signals for SAR. Make your presence known. The universal distress signal in the United States is a grouping of three. It may be three signal fires built in a triangle, three piles of rocks or clothing, three blasts from a whistle, etc. The ideal location is an open area that can be seen from a distance such as a bare hilltop or large clearing. Here are a few options for signaling:

- **Signal fires.** The smoke from a fire can be seen in the daytime and the flames can be seen at night. To increase the smokiness, add green pine needles or leaves.
- **Clothing arranged in an "X."** Bright clothing can be seen from a long distance. If you have an abundance, leave a clothing "X" in a clearing near your shelter.
- **Signal mirror.** I don't usually carry a mirror when running, but they are a great signal device.
- **Rocks, logs, or dirt arranged in the shape of messages.** Use whatever you have available to create notes in open areas. Write the letters "SOS" if possible; otherwise, arrange three piles in a straight line or a triangle. If you move, also include an arrow pointing toward your direction of travel.
- **If you see or hear an aircraft, find an open area and *lie flat on the ground* with your arms and legs spread.** The goal is to be as noticeable as possible.

Step 4: Procure water. After exposure, dehydration is the next danger. Humans can live about three days without water. If you have water, use that. Some people recommend rationing, others suggest drinking normally. There are merits to both approaches. I prefer to ration because it's psychologically demoralizing to run out of water. Regardless of the approach, it's important to avoid heavy exertion. Sweating wastes water.

I discuss methods to find water in an earlier section, including methods to purify potentially dangerous water. Drinking untreated water has risks ranging from illness to death. If you've exhausted your water and are in danger of dehydration, it may be worth the risk of drinking untreated water. Most illnesses may take a week or more before symptoms show up. If people are searching for you and you followed all the advice in here, you'll be found before it becomes an issue.

Step 5: Find food. Food is the last step because humans can survive for weeks without food. While it may seem like an immediate concern, the other steps are *far* more important. If you're trapped in the wilderness long enough to starve, you probably didn't tell someone when or where you were running. Even then, it's unlikely that you would have remained missing.

If you *do* need food, being familiar with local flora and fauna will help. As a general rule of thumb, most furry mammals can be eaten, as well as snakes (cut the head off far enough back to remove poison sacs on poisonous species), fish, and insects that aren't furry, or brightly colored, or those that sting. Plants are more of a mixed bag. Some are okay; others will make you sick. Some will kill. It's best to consult a field guide specific to your area for better information. Or use Google—it's quicker.

These steps constitute the most basic of survival tactics, but nothing can replace field experience. If you plan on spending a lot of time in the backcountry, a survival course taught by qualified instructors can be an awesome addition to your knowledge base.

FIRST AID KIT

In the event you experience any sort of emergency, a first aid kit can literally be a lifesaver. Unfortunately, survival gear takes up a lot of room. Unlike hikers, runners have to be judicious about the gear they carry. What I decide to carry is heavily dependent on local conditions. Trail runs through the relatively safe Michigan countryside aren't nearly as dangerous as backcountry mountain trails. Weather also plays a role. Cold, heat, precipitation, and the availability of shelter factor into the decision of what to carry.

If I'm close to civilization and running on popular, safe trails, I usually don't carry anything. If I'm doing a longer run in a relatively safe environment, I may bring foot care provisions like a few band-aids, alcohol wipes (for sterilization), a safety pin (to lance blisters or remove slivers), and super glue (to close minor wounds).

If I'm running in adverse conditions that could present a danger or I'm traveling further from civilization, I may carry:

- A butane lighter for fire starting
- A space blanket for makeshift shelters, heat reflector, solar still, cord (if cut in strips), or emergency signaling device

- A small, sharp pocket knife
- A plastic poncho or garbage bag if rain is in the forecast
- A flashlight with fresh batteries
- A few meters of parachute cord
- An emergency whistle

These basic items can be used to build a shelter and build a fire. All these items together take up about as much space and weigh as much as two decks of playing cards and can be carried in a hydration pack, fanny pack (for those who want to channel the early 1990s), or water bottle pockets. I've even attached some of that gear to a wide-brimmed straw gardener's hat.

SURVIVAL STUFF

Survival skills are great to learn. Unfortunately, a comprehensive explanation of advanced wilderness survival goes way beyond the scope of this book. I will, however, share a few of my favorite tips.

In the Cold

Cold weather presents two distinct dangers: losing extremities due to frostbite and dying from hypothermia.

Frostbite occurs when blood stops flowing to a region because of cold-induced vasoconstriction. To prevent frostbite, cover up. A layer of clothing over exposed skin usually prevents frostbite when moving. If you stop, make sure you keep everything covered and as dry as possible. If an area starts to hurt due to cold, warm it slowly. Fingers can be placed against your body (I like armpits). For toes, use a friend's armpits if available. If your face is freezing, bury it in a friend's chest—I use that line on Shelly a lot. If you're alone, build a fire. If you can't build a fire, warm your hands and then apply them to the affected area. Repeat as necessary.

Hypothermia is a bigger danger to life. Part of the problem is judgment. When hypothermia begins to set in, people do really stupid stuff like strip off all their clothes. To prevent hypothermia, stay dry and warm; moving usually generates enough heat to maintain body temperature, which is the reason we see so few ultrarunning alligators. You know, they're cold blooded and all.

Anyway, problems usually arise when you're drenched in sweat or fall through ice. If this happens, act immediately. It's usually better to keep clothing on. If you have the capability to build a fire, do so immediately. If not, try to keep moving toward safety. If neither option is available, building shelter may provide a degree of protection from the cold. The wind is usually the killer—if you can effectively block the wind, your chances of survival increase dramatically. If you do build a snow shelter, remember to leave a breathing hole and provide insulation between your body and the snowy walls and floor. If you're with a group, huddle together. The shared body heat can be enough to ward off hypothermia.

In the Heat

Getting too hot presents the same dangers as being too cold, just in the opposite direction. Hyperthermia is a significant danger for runners. Our bodies do a great job of cooling . . . to a point. In the thermoregulation chapter, I place some of the blame on runners overheating by wearing moisture-wicking clothing in hot, dry weather.

Many ultrarunners erroneously believe that consuming adequate fluids and electrolytes will solve the overheating problem. I call bullshit. If we outpace the body's ability to cool off, we'll develop hyperthermia and could die.

The solution is simple: *stop running when you get too hot.* When you stop moving, you stop generating heat. This process can be aided by seeking shade and dousing your skin or clothing with water. This can be effective because you can use any water source, even if it's polluted. Got a urine fetish? Here's your chance to publicly indulge without fear of social rejection. Who can pass judgment when lives are at stake?

BUILDING A FIRE

In the event you're lost or injured, the ability to build a fire could mean the difference between life or death. It can be used for warmth, cooking, signaling, or warding off dangerous animals. Whenever I venture into the backcountry, I always prepare for the possibility of having to build a fire. I've tried several primitive methods of fire-starting, and quite frankly, it's hard. *Really hard.* Instead of pissing with rocks or bows, I carry a simple Bic butane lighter. It is lightweight, reliable, and waterproof. A new lighter could feasibly be used for several weeks of daily fire-starting.

The first step is to find an adequate location for the fire. The purpose of the fire will partially determine location. Ideally, look for a flat, relatively open area free of flammable materials. Flat rocks or bare earth are good choices. A dry, grassy field is a not a good choice. Rocks can be used to construct a fire ring which will help contain the fire.

Types of Fires

There are a variety of designs that will serve different purposes. Knowing a few basics will increase the efficiency of the fires. Here are the ones I use:

- **Teepee fires:** The fuel for teepee fires is arranged in a pyramid or teepee shape. This fire allows a great deal of oxygen to circulate, producing a hot fire that burns quickly. This is my preferred fire for most occasions, including "let's head out to the wilderness, build a fire, get naked, and drink beer" fires.
- **Log cabin fire:** This fire utilizes horizontal pieces laid in a square alternating from side to side with the initial fire built in the middle. This type of fire doesn't emit as much heat, but lasts longer and provides a flat surface for cooking.
- **Star fire:** A small teepee is built in the middle, then five timbers are placed flat on the ground in the shape of a star. One end is touching the teepee. As the fire burns, the timbers are pushed into the center for fuel. This fire lasts a long time and can also provide a decent surface for cooking.

- **Trench fire:** This fire is ideal for windy conditions. A 12" x 36" x 12" deep trench is dug running parallel to the prevailing wind. The wind will create a draft to fuel the fire while still providing enough protection to start it. Line the trench with rocks to help radiate heat upward. A fire is built in the middle of the trench. I like to use a teepee design. The trench can also be used to support cookware or skewers.

Starting and Maintaining the Fire

Getting that initial flame is the tough part. The rest is a matter of understanding the basic principles of fire. To build a fire, two things are needed: fuel and oxygen. The fuel can be pretty much anything flammable. Oxygen is obviously present in the air we breathe, but can be enhanced by blowing on flames or building the fire to use wind to provide greater oxygen flow.

First, the fuel issue. When building a fire, start with small flammable materials that have a lot of surface area. This is known as *tinder*. Good tinder could be lint from your belly button, dry pine needles, dry grass, paper, the fluffy fibers from cattails, dry moss, potato chips, nuts, dry leaves, and steel wool. Many runners carry petroleum-based lube or lip balm, both of which can be used to coat tinder to make it burn better. Pine sap can be used in the same way.

Once the tinder is lit, *kindling* can be added. This should be made up of flammable materials slightly larger than the tinder. Small, dry sticks work great. Once they begin to burn, progressively larger timbers can be added as fuel. Some designs, like the log cabin fire, will already have the fuel built into the design. Others, like the teepee, will require fuel to be added. The star design will require the timbers to be pushed toward the center.

Size Matters

The fire should be just large enough to serve the intended purpose. Novices tend to channel their inner teenager and make fires too big, which wastes fuel and increases the danger of igniting the surrounding environment. Start with a small fire, then increase the size as needed. It's easier to increase size than it is to decrease it.

GPS

Global positioning system (GPS) technology is a marvel of the modern world. By using a series of geostationary satellites coupled with receivers here on Earth, we can find our exact location anywhere. It allows us to get directions and track mileage, our route, and our velocity.

The most common devices used by runners are basically wristwatches. They collect data as we move, which is then uploaded to a computer for analysis and sharing.

This data can be used for a variety of purposes. I like to know the speed, distance, and elevation change of the routes I run. It also provides a cool compilation of your travels. Shelly and I saved the data from our runs as we traveled the country. This has been useful when recommending specific trails to others.

Most road runners fall in love with their GPS watches because the data can be endlessly analyzed. Trail runners seem to either love or hate them. The data can be great, but obsessing over your pace or distance may distract you from enjoying the natural surroundings that define trail running.

GPS devices can serve as useful rescue tools for trail runners. If you become lost or injured and have a means of communicating (cell phone, for example), a GPS device can give your exact location, which can be relayed to search and rescue (SAR) personnel. Also, most devices have a "return to start" function that allows you to backtrack your path or return via a direct line. I've had to use this function on more than one occasion when running in unfamiliar areas.

MAP AND COMPASS

A map and compass are basic necessities for hikers, but most runners leave them at home. A decent topographical map and compass take up a lot of room and most runners simply rely on knowledge of the area or trail markings for navigation.

But what if you're venturing into unknown or poorlymarked areas? Carrying a map and compass becomes a critical necessity. Getting lost in the backcountry is not only dangerous but it taxes rescue resources and puts others at risk. It tends to be expensive, too.

The first step is acquiring the right map. The best maps tend to be topographical maps produced by the US Geological Society (USGS) or private companies that produce more detailed maps based off the USGS maps. They will list most trails, roads, water, and have accurate elevation profiles denoted with shading and contour lines. These maps can be purchased at local outdoor stores or bookstores. The maps are easy to decipher with the legend.

Any basic compass can be used to determine magnetic north. This, in conjunction with an accurate map, can be used to determine your location on most maps by comparing your surroundings to the landforms on the map. This very rudimentary method is about as advanced as I get when using a map and compass in the field.

For those who are more detail oriented, a good map and compass can be used for intricate navigation, including adjusting for the difference between magnetic and true north, navigating from one landmark to another, and finding your exact location using triangulation from visible landmarks. The exact details of these skills go beyond the scope of this book, but are easy to learn via the Internet or classes offered by companies like REI.

In other words, most trail runners don't give a damn about learning intricate navigation skills and carrying the requisite tools. *We're stupid that way.*

NATURAL NAVIGATION AIDS

In the event you don't have a compass and map, it's still possible to ascertain direction using a few natural methods, including:

- **The sun:** It rises in the east and sets in the west. It doesn't get much more basic than that.

- **Stick shadow method:** Place a stick in the ground, then place a pebble at the end of the shadow. Wait about thirty minutes. Place another pebble at the end of the second shadow. Draw a line between the pebbles. The first pebble is west, the second is east. North is perpendicular to the line in the direction away from the stick.
- **North Star:** In the Northern Hemisphere, you can find north by locating the North Star. Look for the Big Dipper constellation. The far edge of the ladle (the right end of the constellation) points toward the North Star, which is five times the distance from the edge of the ladle to the North Star.
- **Snow:** Snow will first melt on the southern-facing slopes in the Northern Hemisphere.
- **Moss:** This tends to be unreliable, but moss usually grows more on the shadowy north side of any object in the Northern Hemisphere.
- **Satellite dishes:** Okay, this isn't quite "natural," but nonetheless it is effective. If you see a house with a satellite dish, the dish will always point south in the Northern Hemisphere.

CELL PHONES

If you are running in an area with reception, a cell phone can be a potential lifesaver. Get lost? Call Search and Rescue. Get hurt? Call for an extraction. Get bored? Play Angry Birds.

However, cell phones are only effective if your battery lasts throughout the trip and you're in a place with adequate reception. Many remote trails in the United States are far from cell towers, so phones are useless. There are products on the market like boosters, repeaters, and directional antennas, which can be used to increase the range of a cell phone, but they're not practical to carry while running.

Since I tend to run in many areas with poor reception, I rarely carry a phone. If I do, I keep it in "airplane mode" unless needed. If left in regular mode, the phone will actively send out signals to establish a connection with towers in the area, which will drain the battery faster. (Thanks to James Barstad for that tip.)

If you plan on carrying your cell phone on a regular basis, invest in a waterproof case. Sweat, rain, snow, and water crossings can destroy your phone after a single exposure. I've had to learn this lesson the hard way . . . twice. The first incident occurred when I ran through a series of lawn sprinklers (I was cutting through the yard of a local church to avoid a road). The second came when I carried my phone in my hydration pack pocket adjacent to my body. The sweat soaked through my shirt and the pack material. The lesson: if you're going to carry a cell phone when trail running, it's a good idea to purchase the insurance.

PERSONAL LOCATION BEACONS

Personal Location Beacons (PLB) are small devices designed to assist search and rescue units by alerting them of an emergency and giving them your location. Some devices (the better choice) use a 406 MHz signal relayed by satellite. Other options, like the SPOT emergency beacon, use similar methods. All devices work by sending a distress signal to a central location where the signal is forwarded to local authorities. When the unit is purchased, a registration is submitted that gives SAR valuable information such as your name, contact phone numbers, etc. Once a signal is received, a rescue team will be dispatched.

Since these devices do not rely on cell phone signals, they can be invaluable in remote locations. The technology is reliable and accurate. The only real downside is false alarms. Many rescue outfits have responded to nonemergency situations (like campers being too cold), which is a monumental waste of resources. If you use a PLB, make sure it's only used in a genuine emergency.

PERSONAL PROTECTION

Sometimes trail running will bring you to dangerous locations. That danger may come from animals or other people. Because of this, some people prefer to carry some sort of personal protection. Some common choices are mace, pepper spray, knives, kubotan, or even guns. Never know when you'll wanna cap an ass out in the boonies!

Of these choices, pepper spray would probably be the most effective as a deterrent. Not only could it be used against people but it could also be used against bears, wolves, or mountain lions. If you don't have pepper spray, hot sauce can be used in a pinch. Of course, the effective range is dramatically reduced. If an attacker confronts you with a "Give me your damn money!" request, you're forced to respond with "How about a nice facial massage instead?" The rest of the choices are rather cumbersome, though I do carry a small pocket knife and flashlight on very long backcountry trail runs.

The key to all options is knowing how to use the weapon. In the unlikely event you'll need to use the weapon, you probably won't have much warning. In short, practice with the weapon. Know how to use it and carry it in a way that it can be utilized immediately. Pepper spray doesn't do much good against an attacking grizzly if you have to dig it out of the bottom of your hydration pack.

As I've mentioned before, both Shelly and I have started training at a mixed martial arts gym, where we're learning boxing, kickboxing, and jujitsu fighting techniques. Who knows, they may come in handy if we're attacked on a trail. I doubt we'll be able to choke out a cougar or grizzly bear, but it *does* boost confidence.

FAMILIARITY WITH LOCAL WEATHER PATTERNS

Pretty much everywhere Shelly and I traveled, we encountered the phrase, "If you don't like the weather here in [insert state here], wait fifteen minutes." While it's true some areas of the country have truly unpredictable weather, most weather patterns can be divined hours or even days ahead of time. As a general rule, weather patterns in North America usually move from west to east. Look west. Whatever weather you see will hit you in the near future. Temperature and humidity (along with a few other factors) can be used in conjunction with the time of year to get a reliable snapshot of possible weather patterns.

As an example, late afternoon thunderstorms during the hot summer days are a predictable pattern for the Colorado Rocky Mountains. If you're familiar with that almost-daily occurrence, you'll avoid summiting mountains in the afternoon (unlike Shelly and I when we summited a 14er just as the afternoon thunderstorms developed . . . took days to clean my shorts).

Before running in a new area, take a few minutes to check local hiking guides or the local weather service's website. They will give you tips on the expected weather conditions for that season.

CHECKING THE WEATHER FORECAST

Once you're familiar with local weather patterns, you'll know what you can reasonably expect as a worst-case scenario. Checking the immediate forecast will give you exact details of what to expect. Well, as exact as meteorology can be.

Prior to any running excursion, I'll check *www.wunderground. com* and at least one local news outlet to get the weather forecast. I look at the hourly forecasts to determine temperatures and the likelihood of precipitation. I also look at the five-day forecast and pay special attention to overnight low temperatures. In the unlikely event I get lost and am forced to spend a night or two in the wilderness, I like to know just how bad it will get. *This forecast always dictates the gear and clothing I'll carry.*

NATURAL WEATHER PREDICTORS

Learning natural weather predictors is a great tool to add to your repertoire of knowledge. If you forget to check the local forecast, nature provides more than enough clues to predict the weather hours or even days before the shit hits the fan.

Clouds

Clouds are among the most reliable predictors of weather . . . mostly because they are the source of precipitation. Here are the common types:

- **Cirrostratus** - These high, wispy clouds are a sign of good weather in the immediate future, but precipitation may be on the way in twelve to twenty-four hours.
- **Stratocumulus** - These clouds appear as big lumpy clouds that cover most of the sky. They generally indicate no weather change in the near future.
- **Cumulonimbus** - These are the giant, tall clouds that look a little bit like an anvil. These clouds are

bad. They produce thunderstorms. If you see them approaching, seek cover.

- **Stratus** - These clouds form an even sheet across the entire sky. They usually produce long-lasting light rain or drizzle.
- **Cumulus** - These are the clouds that look like cotton balls. If they're spread far apart and are relatively small, they represent fair weather. If they are beginning to grow in size vertically, that's an indicator of approaching storms.

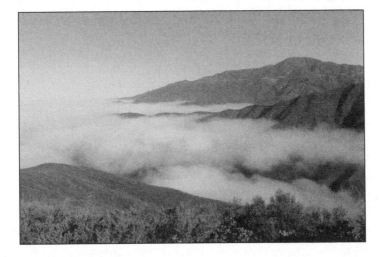

Red Skies

"Red sky at night, sailors' delight. Red sky in the morning, sailors take warning."

I first heard this saying on the elementary school playground in second grade. I thought it was dumb. How could the color of the sky actually predict rain? As it turns out, the saying is a moderately accurate measure of upcoming weather, as long as you're not in the tropics or polar circles. I took a weather class as a freshman at Central Michigan University. The prof gave a lengthy explanation of the phenomenon.

The concept is based on particles in the air. The setting sun turns the westerly sky red at sunset if there's a lot of dust particles in the air, which is synonymous with high pressure. High pressure usually indicate calm weather. Since weather systems generally move west to east, the high pressure will predominate the following day. It could also be caused by a lack of westerly clouds in the sky (since the clouds would block out the sunset).

The red sky in the morning phenomenon is attributed to a few things. First, it could be high particle content from an already-passed system, which means low pressure is near. It could also be caused by clear skies to the east, which is an indicator of an already-passed high pressure system.

Calm before the Storm

Sometimes violent weather can be preceded by an eerie "calm" where the wind dies down and everything seems to get quiet. This occasional phenomenon is a bad sign—a storm is imminent. Not all storms produce this calm period, so don't use this as your lone predictive method.

The "calm" is caused by a vacuum created when a storm sucks warm, moist air into the center of the low pressure cell. This sucking can suck air from all directions, including ahead of the storm. As the air circulates through the clouds, moisture is removed as temperatures drop. The now dry, stable air spills out over the storm and back to your location. The result is the calm before the storm.

The problem with this predictor is timing—it usually occurs within five to fifteen minutes before a storm hits. In fact, it's common to hear the rumble of thunder or see the storm clouds to the west well before you experience the calm. By the time you feel the calm, you have precious little time to take cover.

Pine Cones

Pine cones are nature's hygrometer. In humid conditions, pine cones expand. In dry conditions, they contract. Generally speaking, high humidity precedes wet weather, and low humidity precedes dry weather.

Wind Direction

Wind direction can be used to predict weather patterns. If there's a westerly wind, there's a good chance the weather is going to be fair. If there's an easterly wind, it's a sign the weather is about to change for the worst.

This one has to do with the nature of low-pressure systems, which are associated with storms. The low-pressure system swirls counter-clockwise. As it approaches an area, this counter-clockwise rotation causes the wind to shift from the west to the east.

Cows

When I was a kid, I grew up in close proximity to a dairy farm. I spent a good portion of my youth around cows. It was magical. If you happen to have access to cows, they can be used as a minimally reliable makeshift weather vane. Cows have a weird peculiarity:

they prefer to have wind blowing at their asses versus their heads. As such, they tend to stand away from the prevailing wind. Based on the idea above, if cows are facing east, expect good weather. If cows are facing west, expect bad weather. Weird, huh?

Campfires

When a high-pressure system is present, the air is stable. When a low-pressure system is present, the air is turbulent. If you build a campfire, the behavior of the smoke can indicate high or low pressure. If the smoke rises straight up or is carried in one direction, it's likely due to the stability of high pressure. Expect good weather in the near future. If the smoke swirls unpredictably, it's likely due to the turbulence of low pressure. Expect bad weather.

Frizzy or Curly Hair

Hair out of control? It could be the result of high humidity, which is a sign of precipitation in the near future. I have Shelly to thank for this one. As we travel, we routinely visit areas with higher or lower humidity. She'll often comment about the effects of the area on her hair. The key is waiting for her hair to suddenly get curly in an area where it was otherwise relatively flat. That's a sign rain is in the forecast.

Bugs

In many areas, insects can be used to predict weather. I find ants to be among the most reliable. If rain is near, ants tend to flee back to their nests. If you see a lot of ants moving in the same direction, it's probably going to rain soon. Ants also build the domes at the entrance to their nests higher and will cap them off prior to rain.

Biting insects usually bite more often immediately prior to rain. In Michigan, we could predict rain by the increased aggressiveness of black flies (late spring) and deer flies (summer). I've been told the same rules apply in other geographic areas.

Dew on Grass

If there's dew on the grass in the morning, it's a good sign fair weather is in the immediate forecast. If the grass is dry, expect precipitation. This concept has to do with wind. Dew only forms in relatively calm conditions associated with high pressure. If there's a low-pressure front approaching, the winds will pick up and prevent dew from forming.

Speaking of dew—if you ever need an emergency water source, drag a piece of fabric over dew-covered grass, then wring it out over a container. It's possible to collect enough water to satisfy your daily needs.

Jet Tails

Jet tails are the condensed water trails left by jets as they pass overhead, which are sometimes known as contrails. Jet tails normally dissipate within a minute or so. Higher moisture content in the air will increase their longevity. If they last significantly longer, there could be precipitation within a day.

Moon Rings

Rings that appear around the moon can also be used to predict weather. The rings are caused by high-altitude ice particles, which precede precipitation.

WHAT TO DO IN A SEVERE THUNDERSTORM

In the event you're stuck outdoors in a severe storm, a few steps will keep you safe. The key is to protect yourself from lightning, flood waters, and hail.

Know when to seek cover. The distance of an approaching storm can be determined by the differential between seeing the light of the lightning and hearing the sound of the thunder. Count the number of seconds between the lightning and thunder, then divide by five. That will give you the distance in miles. If you're more of a metric system fan, divide by three for kilometers. Since lightning can strike miles ahead of the storm clouds, you should seek cover when the lightning and thunder are separated by thirty seconds or less.

If you're in an open area or a place with a variety of elevations, move away from high ground. Get off summits and ridges. However, don't go too low. Low areas are prone to flash flooding, so avoid the bottom of valleys or channels. You can usually determine floodplains by a noticeable debris line. Stay away from lone trees or other tall, solitary objects. If you're in a group, separate by at least twenty-five feet. This will prevent the entire group from being struck by a single lightning strike.

Hail can be dangerous if it's larger than a dime. If it begins to hail, take cover under a sturdy object like a cave, rock outcropping, or a fallen tree. If you don't have sturdy cover, drop to your knees, place your head near the ground, and cover it with your hands or any other object you're carrying. The goal is to avoid head trauma.

LEARNING TO FALL

Huh? Isn't falling, by definition, something you can't predict?

Yes. But you can develop your ability to fall *better*.

Falling while trail running is inevitable. Most people do their best to avoid falling and hope they don't get hurt too badly if the unfortunate happens. I'm clumsy. I don't like to take those chances.

So how do you go about learning to fall?

Find a location with soft ground. Sand is perfect. Grassy fields are another good choice. Run at a slow speed, then purposely fall on the ground. I prefer to use a "slow your fall with your arms, then roll" technique. As you're falling, keep your elbows bent. When you hit the ground with your hands, the bent elbows will act as shock absorbers. Locked elbows can cause a "FOOSH" injury: falling on out-stretched hands. The impact can shatter all bones of the arm, which is not pretty. As my arms are absorbing the shock, I begin rolling my body to the side away from the most dangerous debris. Depending on the trail, I may roll several times.

This specific technique will not work on all trails. For example, it may be impossible to avoid serious injury if falling on rocky mountain trails. In that case, do what you can to avoid smacking your head on a sharp rock. *Protect your head at all costs!* I prefer to carry handheld water bottles to help soften the blow of landing hard on my hands. The bottles usually take a beating, but it saves my hands. Wearing gloves can also serve the same purpose, but may be too hot depending on the weather.

If you're searching for more training on the proper way to fall, grappling training (wrestling, jiujitsu, or judo) is useful as it teaches body position, balance, and methods to dissipate the force of falling (known as "break falling"). I've also been told sky divers are pretty good at falling. If any of these things are on your bucket list, it could be a nice "two birds" sort of deal.

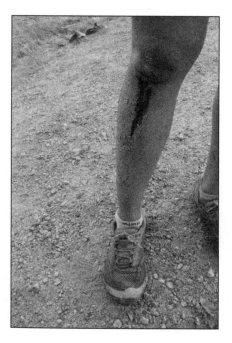

FALLING OFF A CLIFF

Full disclaimer: I've never fallen off a cliff. However, I have run in many environments where it was a distinct possibility. A few years ago, I met a dude on a trail that gave me some *"Oh shit!"* advice, including what to do if you fall off a cliff. His first bit of wisdom: *Don't fall off a cliff.* His second bit of wisdom: *It's not the fall that's bad; it's the landing.*

Eventually he got around to actual useful advice.

The trick to falling is learning to land in a way that dissipates as much energy as possible. Try to land on your feet. As soon as you touch the ground, roll forward in a ball. If done correctly, this redirects a significant amount of energy. It's possible to practice the technique by jumping off a raised platform. Start with something low . . . maybe a foot off the ground and progress to higher platforms as you develop the skill.

If you're sliding down a steep hill, you can usually stop the falling using friction. Roll to your belly and spread your arms and legs. It's like doing a face-down gravel angel.

DANGEROUS FAUNA

Sometimes trail runners encounter animals. Sometimes those animals can hurt you. Most are easy to handle . . . *if you know how to react.* Here's a rundown of the most common animals encountered in North America.

Snakes

Before running in a new area, learn to identify the native poisonous snakes. Should you encounter one on the trail, avoid it. Furthermore, avoid putting your hands and feet in areas you cannot see. As a general rule, snakes can strike better when coiled versus stretched across the trail.

If you are bitten, stay in one place if others will be passing (like a race). Otherwise, get to safety as quickly as possible. Evacuation via helicopter or motor vehicle is best, followed by walking. Running will cause your heart to beat faster, which circulates the venom faster. Restrict movement as much as possible, which can include splinting the affected area. Try to identify the snake, but don't risk others being bitten. If it helps, only a fraction of 1 percent of snakebite victims actually die from the bite.

Spiders and Scorpions

Spiders and scorpions present many of the same dangers as snakes—they may be venomous. Learn to identify the really dangerous species in your area. If you are bitten or stung, follow the same guidelines.

A major difference between snakes and spiders/scorpions has to do with clothing—spiders and scorpions may crawl into your clothing or shoes and will bite you when dressing. Not only is the experience traumatic but you'll likely have nightmares for decades. It's good to get in the habit of shaking out your clothing and shoes before putting them on.

Bees and Wasps

Bees and wasps aren't usually as dangerous . . . unless you have an allergy to their venom. If you *are* allergic to bee venom, it's a good idea to carry an epinephrine pen when trail running.

If you are stung, escape the area. Avoid that particular area as the bees or wasps will probably be agitated. Odds are good you disrupted their nest. If the stinger is stuck in your skin, scrape it off with your fingernail.

While running the Burning River hundred-miler a few years ago, I stepped on a wasp nest. I was only stung on the heel (I was wearing huarache sandals) and thigh. The next ten miles sucked before the pain dissipated, but I was lucky. I was wearing a kilt for the race. The thoughts of getting stung in the junk was enough to dissuade me from wearing a kilt for any future trail race.

Ticks

Ticks are mostly a problem on the East Coast, where they're known to carry Lyme disease. To avoid ticks, stay on the trail.

Avoid long grass immediately off the trail. If you find a tick attached to your skin, remove it with tweezers, wash with soap, and apply antiseptic to the area.

Bears

Most bears in the United States will avoid contact with humans unless they're protecting cubs, territory, or they feel you're threatening their food supply. If you do encounter a bear and it isn't aware of your presence, back away slowly. If it is aware of your presence, make some noise and talk in a low voice. Avoid eye contact. The goal is to identify yourself as a human. The bear will probably try to avoid you.

If a bear does attack, don't run. They have no problem outrunning a human. The only situation where running is advisable: your running partner is both annoying *and* slower than you. Otherwise, climb a high tree if possible. Note: black bears are good climbers. Unless you can get to branches that will support your weight but not their weight, climbing is futile.

If you have pepper spray, this is the time to use it. Spray it before the bear actually reaches you.

If they make physical contact, you're in trouble. There are two schools of thought—fight back or play dead. Since many bear attacks are defensive in nature, they will stop when they believe the threat has been neutralized. Personally, I'd play dead. If you *do* decide to fight back, having a weapon helps.

Moose, Elk, and Deer

Most people don't concern themselves with these seemingly peace-loving herbivores. However, they can and will attack humans and are capable of killing.

Like with bears, keep your distance. Announce your presence. If they charge, get behind cover to separate yourself from them. Trees or large rocks work well. If they do reach you, fall to the ground, cover your head, and play dead. They will probably stop stomping you once they believe the threat is neutralized.

Cougars

Cougars, at least in the western United States, present a real threat. They are adept predators, and they have an uncanny ability to stalk their prey. Once they determine you're a target, you're essentially powerless. The trick is to be able to identify their presence. In my experience, the easiest way to detect cougars is through the smell of their perfume and the clicking of high heels. . . .

Yes, that may be the worst joke in the entire book. I'm *almost* embarrassed for including it.

Older women preying on younger men aside, mountain lions can be scary because their presence will rarely be known until they're actually attacking you. If you do see a mountain lion, make eye contact. Raise your arms. Appear as big as possible. Make noise. Act aggressive. The big cat is looking for an easy kill, not a protracted fight.

If they *do* attack, don't turn your back. If you have children with you, pick them up. If you value your kids, it will protect them from the cougar's attach. If you don't, they make handy, though noisy, shields. Use sticks, rocks, running gear, or your fists as weapons. Aim for their eyes, nose, or throat. The goal is to convince the cougar you're a threat and not worth the fight.

RUNNING DURING HUNTING SEASON

I grew up in a small northern Michigan rural community. Hunting was part of our DNA. Every fall, 75 percent of the population gathered their small personal arsenals of firearms, loads of ammo, and a six pack of beer and hit the forest in search of rabbit, squirrels, partridge, deer, bear, etc. I have distinct memories of sitting in a deer blind in the predawn darkness as the first hints of color appeared in the eastern sky. The first gunshot caused me to jump a bit because it seemed far too early to see a deer through the darkness. That first shot would be followed by a steady stream of gunshots, usually about one shot every thirty seconds.

I also remember thinking how ridiculously dangerous this was—thousands of hunters of questionable sobriety armed with the same rifles used by military snipers shooting at anything that moved. I'm still amazed the number of accidental shootings was as low as it was.

When I started serious trail running, autumn brought mixed feelings. I loved running through the forest as the leaves were transforming to the brilliant shades of yellow, orange, and red. The sweet smell of fallen leaves filling my nostrils, the chilly air on my face . . . it was magical. Because of the hunters, it was also slightly terrifying. The previous hunting experience helped give a little peace of mind because I could guess where the hunters may be. Still, many of my favorite trails were run through popular hunting areas.

My best advice would be to avoid trails during the most popular hunting seasons. In Michigan, that would be firearm deer season. It may vary in other areas of the country. If you absolutely have to run during hunting season, dress in blaze orange. If any body part isn't covered in blaze orange, it should be covered in dark green or black. Avoid brown, white, or other colors of the local wildlife (I've known too many crazy-ass hunters that shot as soon as they saw a flash of white, the color of a whitetail deer's tail). If you see a hunter, stay several hundred yards away. Better yet, turn around. In all likelihood, your presence will *not* be welcomed by hunters because you're frightening their game. Some hunters, probably the same that shoot without properly identifying their target, have been known to assault nonhunters that encroach in their territory. Public use rules aren't going to stop insane hunters from shooting you, so proceed with extreme caution.

HALLUCINATION

The DNF at Burning River in 2008 was difficult. I was forced to come to terms with the fact that I may not be tough enough to reach the goal. It was similar to the very first year I tried running a fifty-miler but had to settle for the marathon instead. Only worse. At least the previous experience resulted in a finish.

It was painfully apparent my Crossfit and Crossfit Endurance training was only partially effective. I needed the long runs to both increase my physiological capability to run a long distance and to experiment with gear, foods, clothing, etc. Prior to Burning River, I had only run a marathon distance or longer four times, all in races. I also knew the speed-oriented workouts of the CF and CFE programs made me a faster, more efficient runner. My new goal was to develop my own hybrid program that incorporated the best of everything I had tried up to that point.

I knew I needed to do long runs. I knew the speedwork and high intensity interval training was good and should be continued. If I could find a balance between the two, I knew I could finish a hundred-miler. For the running element, I created a plan that included several short, fast runs during the week, followed by a long run on the weekend. For the weight training element, I enlisted the help of friend and Crossfit trainer John DeVries. He programmed his own workouts, which deviated significantly from the normal Crossfit workouts of the day. His workouts focused more on the specific muscle groups I'd be using during the race.

Once I had a workout plan, I needed a race. I decided on a brand-new hundred-miler held in Michigan—the Hallucination 100. It was part of a trail running festival called "Run Woodstock" put on by Randy Step of Running Fit, a local running store chain. It was a looped course over hilly, rocky trails.

I spent the entire spring and summer training harder than I ever had before. My body, after several years of heavy training, could better withstand the rigors of high mileage and hard weight training. I was also smart enough to rest when the specter of injuries popped up. I also dialed in my planning. I cut out a lot of the unnecessary crap from the previous year, and assembled a crew and pacers (Jason Saint Amour, Shelly, Mark Robillard, Stuart Peterson, and Michael Helton). By the end of summer, I was ready.

I wrote a lengthy race report of this particular race in *The Barefoot Running Book*, so I'll spare the excessive details. It hurt, and I supposedly hallucinated about killer bees for the last few miles, but I finished. The race proved to be a great learning experience. Some highlights:

- Chia seeds, no matter how much they're promoted in *Born to Run*, make a terrible ultramarathon food. Five pounds of those devil seeds contain a criminal amount of fiber. I might as well have eaten ExLax and bird shit as a race food.

- Vibram Five Fingers probably aren't the best shoe for hundred-milers. Yes, they allow for great "ground feel." No, I *do not* want to feel every single rock, root, and acorn for one hundred miles.
- It helps immensely to have a pacer that is wellversed in show tunes. Stuart Peterson's sweet voice carried me through some dark miles toward the end.
- Ultras hurt. Unfortunately, the hurt doesn't stop when you cross the finish line. I have vague, sleep-derived memories of being handed a buckle, limping across a grassy field, sitting in a lawn chair, eating a hot dog, and drinking a beer. I expected to be filled with pride as I finally reached this pinnacle I dreamed about years earlier. Instead, I was just relieved to have this whole damned "ultrarunning" thing behind me.

SECTION 5:
ULTRARUNNING BASICS

ULTRAMARATHONS!

Why You Should Run Ultras

Prize money? No. Even if you win, the winnings probably won't even pay for the food you ate during the race. *Fame?* Nope. People will think you're crazy . . . and not "the party doesn't start until you arrive" kind of crazy. *Health?* Not even close. I usually feel about twenty years older *after* finishing a race.

So why bother? It comes down to one simple fact: you'll never be this young again. There's nothing more empowering than completing a race 99.99 percent of the human population would never even consider, let alone attempt. You'll forever compare an ultra finish to difficult life events. You'll realize you really can accomplish far more than you expect. This empowering experience can be life changing.

Since Shelly and I adopted our hobo lifestyle, we've come across a few tough times. The experience of running hundos has reinforced the idea that I can survive pretty much anything as long as I keep moving forward.

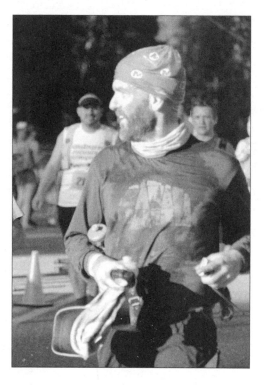

There may be other reasons, too. You get cool swag, like shirts, belt buckles, and beer mugs. You get to experience nature up close and personal. You get to brag to your friends. You can say rude stuff like, "You run marathons? Awwww . . . how cute!" You meet incredible people and bond over your mutual struggles. You get to poop in the woods. And the groupies . . . can't forget the groupies!

Okay, there are no groupies. In fact, the only people that seem to be attracted to sweaty, smelly ultrarunners are, well, other ultrarunners.

Still not convinced? Start hanging out with ultrarunners. Volunteer to work at an aid station for a local race. Google "ultra-marathon race report," then read a few. Crew or pace a friend as they complete an ultra. I guarantee you'll catch the bug!

ARE ULTRAS HEALTHY OR DANGEROUS?

Most experts would recommend moderate exercise as a required component to any healthy lifestyle. Unfortunately, there's nothing moderate about running over potentially dangerous terrain for hours and hours. Acute injuries are part of the game. But what about longer-term injuries?

In 2012, an article was published discussing the potential long-term damage that could occur in some endurance athletes (O'Keefe et al.). The prolonged, heavy blood flow through the heart could do a little bit of scar tissue damage, and this damage could build up over time. The result would be an irregular heartbeat, which could be fatal.

There's no doubt ultras push past the "healthy amount of exercise" threshold. The authors of the study were careful to note excessive exercise, while potentially damaging, was still superior to no exercise at all.

There's little doubt running ultras is a risk, but probably not nearly as risky as a sedentary lifestyle. The heart research hits especially close to home because my father died unexpectedly at a relatively young age due to a heart attack. Still, I'm a firm believer life is meant to be lived. The places I've seen, people I've met, and memories I've created easily outweigh the potential risk I undertook with every training run and race.

Sometimes I think of where I would be had I never taken the "ultra plunge." I'd probably still be a shitty football coach and disillusioned teacher living in a suburban Hell. Instead, I've spent the last few years living a life of adventure. If given the opportunity to travel back in time and change any one decision, I would make the same choices every time. **175**

WHAT DOES IT TAKE TO RUN ULTRAS?

So you're still deciding if you want to tackle the ultramarathon distance. You're intrigued by the idea, but you have doubts. What exactly does it take to run ultras? As it turns out, it's probably not as difficult as one would imagine.

First, it does take some degree of physical fitness. If your goal is to simply finish the race, it is critical that you have the ability to spend a long period of time on your feet. The "time on feet" will likely be a combination of running and walking. How will you know you are ready? I like to use a 50 percent guideline. If you can estimate your finish time in the planned ultra, your training should allow you to spend at least 50 percent of that time on a single long run. For example, let's say you are planning a fifty-mile run. You anticipate finishing in ten hours. You could probably survive the distance if you are able to do a training run of at least five hours. Greater fitness will obviously increase the chances of finishing, but the 50 percent guideline is useful to determine minimal readiness.

Second, completing an ultra takes training. I do have a good friend, Rich Elliott, that attempted a fifty-mile race with a single five kilometer race as his only training. He made it to about twenty-seven miles before he DNFed (did not finish). That was foolish. Brave, but foolish. In my opinion, one can get by with only a few runs per week and still finish an ultra as long as one of the runs is a long run of ever-increasing distance. Since the guide is for the lazy runners like me, I can admit to rarely running more than three or four days per week.

Third, ultrarunners need to be reasonably familiar with the issues they may face when running very long distances. They must be aware of the signs and symptoms of problems and know the appropriate response. In marathon-and-shorter races, most runners can simply run. If an issue arises, you can gut it out to the finish. In an ultra, that is usually impossible. It's awfully hard to gut out a chafed groin for eight hours.

Fourth, ultrarunners need to be mentally tough. Scrappy and stubborn is more important than talented, because you will experience some degree of pain. In all likelihood, you will experience *a lot* of pain. In my first hundred-mile attempt that ultimately resulted in a DNF at around mile sixty-five, I seriously considered diving on rocks to break an arm just to end the suffering of having to continue. Luckily I was too scared... instead I just let the cutoff times catch me and was mercifully pulled from the course. My problem was simple: I hadn't developed very good strategies for dealing with the pain. The second attempt hurt a lot, too, but I practiced much better pain-management strategies.

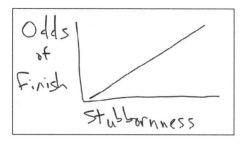

These are what I would consider to be the absolute minimum elements to running an ultra. Other things like prior racing experience, outdoor survival skills, an uncanny ability to navigate through the wilderness, being especially athletically gifted, or single with no children will certainly help. They are not necessities, though. Almost everyone has the ability to run ultras . . . even those that may not believe it today. If you can reasonably master these four elements, you will be in an excellent position to conquer the ultramarathon distances!

Ultras can still be mentally daunting, however. Ultrarunner and motivational speaker Scott Burton (amazingcompanyevents. com) notes most people, when assessing if an ultramarathon is within their abilities, will think "*I can't do that; it's impossible!*" He advises people to think, "*If I gained additional abilities and knowledge, I could do this even if I presently can't.*"

I absolutely love this approach because it removes the easily-accepted excuse we often use when confronted with a difficult task and empowers us to begin the journey toward developing the skill set that will allow us to accomplish the goal. It makes the journey more manageable by breaking ultras down to a set of learned skills, which are accomplished through training. The various topics covered throughout this book provide an excellent guide to the topics you'll need to tackle an ultramarathon.

DON'T YOU HAVE TO BE A GOOD RUNNER?

There's a myth that runners have to be good to run ultramarathons. By "good" I mean fast. Sure, many ultrarunners are blazing fast in shorter races. It's not a prerequisite, though. It's entirely possible to be turtle-slow and still finish an ultra. I would go out on a limb and say it may be advantageous to be slow.

Generally speaking, there's an inverse relationship between speed and distance. As distances increase, speed (as measured by pace) decreases. Once you get to ultra distances, the nonelites are pretty slow. How slow? When I finished my first hundred, my average pace was around 17:30. No, that's not a typo. Yes, most people can walk faster than that. The point . . . it's a *very* slow average pace. Even at my fastest, I doubt I ran more than ten-minute miles.

- In ultras, slow is the name of the game. If you already run slow . . . perfect! You won't have to learn how to restrain yourself in the early miles of ultras. Many novice runners start out way too fast, which results in a severe crash and burn. The ability to run slow is an underappreciated skill set.

- I know you're still doubting me. You've convinced yourself that speed is a necessary ingredient to building long-distance running ability. Unfortunately this belief keeps many runners from ever attempting an ultra. They convince themselves that they have to reach some arbitrary time-based goal at a shorter distance before they can make the jump to ultras. I know people that can run one hundred-plus miles per week, easily drop Boston-qualifying times in marathons, and can recite the ingredients and nutritional value of every energy gel, bar, and drink on the market. Yet they doubt their ability to survive an ultra.

- If your goal is to simply finish (and it should be if this is your first ultra *and* you are truly a lazy runner), pick a goal race . . . maybe a fifty kilometer. Find out the cutoff time (how long you are allowed to finish before everyone packs up and goes home). Go to the cool running pace calculator here: *www.coolrunning.com/engine/4/4_1/96.shtml*. Enter the cutoff time and the distance; it will return your pace. Now go out and run a few miles at that pace.

- *Stop and go run!*

- Okay, now that you're back, how was that pace? Pretty slow, huh? I bet it felt like you weren't even moving. I bet your normal training pace doesn't feel too slow now. That is the minimum you would need to finish the race. Anyone can do that. Don't worry, I'll give you more advice in the coming days . . . just have confidence that your slow running is an asset in ultras!

THE DIFFERENT RACE OPTIONS

The first step to choosing that first ultra is actually choosing the race. The single best resource is *Ultrarunning Magazine*'s online ultra calendar (*www.ultrarunning.com/calendar.html*). The races can be sorted in a variety of ways based on location, distance, difficulty, date, etc. I would recommend starting with distance. There are actually two categories: distance races and timed races. Here are the most common:

- **Fifty kilometers (thirty-one miles):** This is considered the minimum "ultra" distance. It's usually considered to be the easiest. It's a good first choice, especially if you don't want to train for a long period of time.
- **Fifty miles**: This is also a decent choice for a first ultra. It's more difficult, but can still be run in a single day.
- **One hundred kilometers**: This distance is getting into the realm of "too difficult for a first ultra" because it usually requires day and night running.
- **One hundred miles**: Some people start with hundos, but I'd advise against it. You encounter a lot of issues that

are difficult to experience in training. Your best bet is to learn from the shorter distances first.

- **Six hours**: This is probably the shortest timed race where a beginner could reach the ultra distance (50k). The races are usually held on short looped courses with ample aid and other support. However, it would probably require running for the entire six hours, and averaging about an 11:30 minute/mile pace. It is probably better to do a . . .

- **Twelve hours**: This is a great ultra distance to get your feet wet if a 50k is unavailable. Pretty much anybody can reach the ultra distance and still have plenty of time to sit down and rest, eat, and take care of any issues that arise. Think of it as an ultra with training wheels for the newbie. In fact, twelve hours are my favorite race to introduce people to ultra distances. I use simple logic: You can stop at any time, even after one lap.

- **Twenty-four hours**: This is another good option if a twelve hour race isn't available. It can also be a good option for those wanting to train for hundred-milers since it involves night running and sleep deprivation.

- **Forty-eight and Seventy-two hours**: This would be overkill for a newbie . . . no need to go this long unless you're really into adventure!

As if this wasn't enough options, races also come in a few different layouts:

- **Point-to-point:** This race starts at one place and ends at another. Timed races do not use this format. Personally this is my favorite type of race because you don't run on the same part of the course twice. I like the novelty.

For beginners, this is a good choice because you don't come back to the start line, which could give you the opportunity to drop out of the race.

- **Loop:** A looped course is run in a series of, well, loops. All timed races are loop races. Many distance races run in smaller parks are also looped courses. The advantage of loops is course familiarity. Once you run one loop, you've seen all of the course. For some, this is a nice benefit. If you have masochistic friends and family that want to watch you run for the better part of a day, looped courses are ideal.

- **Out-and-back:** These races start at one point, run to another, then run back to the original start line. They have the advantage of course familiarity on the way back, but also make it difficult to stop. Unless you have a rise to the start line, dropping out would still require you to walk all the way back to the start line— the same distance you'd cover if you stayed in the race. Personally, I like to plan training runs as out-and-backs for this very reason.

- **Stage races:** These races are held over the course of a few days. You run a certain distance, rest, then run more the next day. Because of the logistics, these really aren't good "newbie" races . . . and some question if it is actually an ultramarathon if the runners don't cover at least 50k per day.

CHOOSING YOUR FIRST ULTRAMARATHON

If you ask experienced ultrarunners, they will often recommend a specific race as an "ideal first race." Here's the problem: it's the race they recommend *based on their experiences*. Sometimes they're right. Sometimes they're wrong. Their suggestions certainly deserve consideration, but I'd recommend tailoring the choice a little more based on this criteria:

1. **Choose a distance that you can realistically train for given the time frame.** If you're choosing a 50k, a few months will probably be sufficient. A fifty-miler will take more time, as will a 100k or a hundred-miler. You have more latitude with timed races since you can run whatever distance you want.

2. **Pick a race that features terrain and elevation similar to your training grounds.** If you live in Florida where hills are nonexistent, it's probably a bad idea to sign up for a mountain ultra with thousands of feet of climbing and descending. It's the same deal with terrain. Don't sign up for a notoriously rocky ultra if you routinely get passed

by soccer moms pushing jogging strollers on your local trails. The *Ultrarunning* magazine online calendar has a handy one to five rating scale for both terrain and elevation with the higher number representing more elevation and more technical trails.

3. **Bring experienced friends.** Nothing can be more valuable than the support of friends that have ultra experience. When I ran my first ultra, I was helped by a dude that had run several hundred ultras in his lifetime. He ran with me for about twelve miles and kept me from quitting when I hit some serious lows. Since relying on strangers can be difficult, set the stage by asking a friend to run the race side by side with you. If you can't find a willing or experienced friend, join some online ultrarunning communities. It's usually pretty easy to make friends; then ask them for the same favor. If it helps, offer to pay a friend's entry fee.

4. **Don't bite off more than you can chew.** The longer the distance, the more likely issues will arise that will have to be solved. For example, hundred-milers require you to navigate trails in the dark while both fatigued and sleep-deprived. It's difficult to get the needed experience in training. The fewer the variables, the greater your chances of success. You'll have plenty of opportunities to tackle the toughies down the road.

Considering these three issues can go a long way toward finding your "ideal" first ultra. The goal is to put you in a position to succeed, and then use that success to conquer greater challenges in the future.

LEARNING ABOUT THE RACE

Now that you've signed up (and nursed that hangover), you can start researching the intricate details of the race. You'll want to know important things like:

- The race rules
- Lodging options in the area
- Typical weather conditions
- How other runners approached the race

All of these items can be found on the race websites or by reading race reports. When some people run a race, they write race reports to document their experiences. These can be found in a number of places, including ultrarunning forums, blogs, or ultrarunning websites. Some race directors even post race reports on the race website. An easy way to find them is Googling "[insert race name] race report."

Don't discount the best possible resource: runners who have firsthand knowledge of the course or race. If the race is local, it should be pretty easy to find runners who have run the race. Check with local running clubs or running stores.

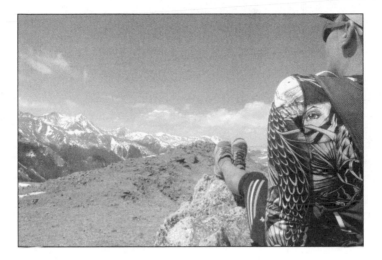

ELEVATION PROFILES

In the last section I mentioned elevation. Most race directors publish what is known as an elevation profile. It's essentially a graph representing how many hills the course has. The "spikier" the graph, the more hills. Also, the steeper the graph, the steeper the hill.

Many recommend a flat course for beginners. Again, I'd recommend picking a course with similar climbs and altitude as your training trails. People who train in the rough stuff usually have some difficulty going to the flat stuff.

If you train at high altitude, you can run a race at lower altitude without problems. Going from low-altitude training to a high-altitude (>8,000 feet) race can be problematic, though. The lower concentration of oxygen can cause altitude sickness. Unless that's your thing. Sure it can be life-threatening, but some people may be into nosebleeds, hangover symptoms, and cerebral edema. To each their own . . . I guess.

Flat Course:

Not So Flat Course:

HOW MUCH DO ULTRAMARATHONS COST?

The price of ultras can range from free to staggeringly expensive. Badwater, a race run through Death Valley in California, can easily cost around $10,000 for the race entry fee, travel, hotels, gear, and rental vehicles. So what is a more realistic price?

Most races range in price from a low of about $30 to a high of about $400. Generally speaking, the longer the race, the more expensive the entry fees. Other variables make a difference, like the level of support offered, the need for permits to use the land, and the swag (goodies like T-shirts and finisher awards).

Aside from the entry fee, other costs need to be considered, including:

- **Transportation**: If the race is within driving distance, you need to consider the price of gas and parking. If the race requires flying, consider airport parking, the cost of the flight, rental car, and gas.

- **Lodging**: Hotels may be needed for the night before and after the race. Hint: always get a room on the first floor. After the race, it will likely be difficult to climb stairs. Some races will offer on-site camping, which can save money. If you camp in a tent, bring plenty of warm blankets. It's not uncommon to feel colder than normal after a race.

- **Food**: You will need food before and after the race, and potentially food during the race. Some races offer pre- and post-race meals. One of the best parts of ultrarunning is that we tend to burn a lot of calories, which means one thing: guilt-free fast food! I recommend Taco Bell. Lay off the spicy sauces, though . . . otherwise you'll regret it the next day. Trust me on this one.

- **Gear**: I prefer to bring as little gear as possible, but it still adds up to a fair amount of crap. I usually bring several clothing options, at least two pair of shoes, sometimes socks (I hate socks), bandana, flashlights and headlamps, lube (prevent chafing), handheld water bottles, and a small foot care kit (I'll discuss that one later). For very long races, I'll also add some more crap to my stockpile. To save money, you can often use nonrunning specific homemade gear. In my first ultra, I used little travel bottles designed for shampoo ($1 each) instead of gel flasks designed for runners ($12 each). Different sections of this book will help you determine what you need to buy.

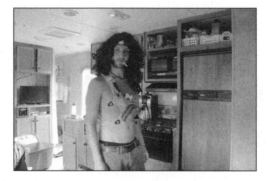

There may be other expenses that arise based on individual experiences. If you use diamond-encrusted GPS watches or eat caviar at the aid stations, the cost is going to be more. For the most part, ultras are pretty cheap compared to other hobbies. The closer you stay to home, the more money you'll likely save on transportation and lodging.

WHAT ABOUT FAT-ASS RACES?

Is this a race for people with giant butts directed by Sir Mix-A-Lot? Not quite. A fat-ass race is essentially an organized "unofficial" race set up by one or a few dedicated ultrarunners. There are no perks (shorts, medals, etc.), course marshals (people who keep you on the course), aid stations or other forms of support, or even a timing mechanism. It's usually more like a training run than a race.

So why would you want to run a fat ass?

They're free!

And they tend to be super cool. The people who show up for fat-ass races are running for the pure love of running and the camaraderie of their fellow runners. I would highly encourage any new ultrarunner to hang out at fat-ass races.

However, I would not recommend a fat-ass as a first race. The lack of support usually requires runners to carry all their food and water, which adds a fairly difficult obstacle to an already big undertaking. Also, the lack of course markings may make the actual course navigation difficult. Again, it's another variable that a brand new ultrarunner shouldn't have to worry about.

THE DIFFERENCE BETWEEN ROAD AND TRAIL ULTRAS

The vast majority of ultras are run on trails of some sort. Some are run on roads. Distance races tend to be more trail oriented, while timed races tend to be more road oriented (which may include things like running tracks or concrete sidewalks through parks).

Is one better than the other?

Not necessarily, though there are significant differences. Road running requires a lot of repetitive motions. Your running gait remains more or less the same for the duration of the event. Furthermore, road races tend to be rather flat. This puts stress on specific sets of muscles, tendons, ligaments, and bones. People like me who train primarily on trails usually have difficulty running on roads.

Most trail runs require the runner to avoid obstacles such as roots, rocks, logs (both wooden and the kind left by animals . . . or lazy humans), and water or mud. Trail races tend to have more elevation change, so you spend more time traversing hills. This requires much more dynamic movement, which distributes the workload to different muscles, tendons, ligaments, and bones. People that train primarily on roads usually have difficulty running on trails.

My suggestion: It's best to choose a race with similar terrain and elevation as your training routes. If you live in a city surrounded by flat farmland, a mountain trail race would be a bad idea. It's the same deal if you like to train on trails with lots of elevation change. A road race will be more difficult than a trail race.

It is possible to take a "jack of all trades" approach and train on both roads and trails, which gives you *much* more versatility. This would be the ideal situation if you have enough time to train before your first ultra.

TAKING THE LEAP AND SIGNING UP

Okay, so you found the perfect race. Now what? I bet you're a little hesitant to register. I have a time-tested method to alleviate that uneasy feeling when you're filling out the registration form. Here's what you need:

- A computer (or mail-in form, envelope, and stamp for those races that are still stuck in the 1900s)
- Credit card (or checkbook)
- A good friend or relative with an antagonistic personality
- Copious amounts of your favorite alcohol

Step 1: Explain the antagonist's role, which is to get you to sign up for the race.

Step 2: Go to the race website registration page.

Step 3: Drink all of the alcohol.

Step 4: Let the antagonist work his or her magic.

Congratulations! You just signed up for your first ultra!

Now tell everyone you know. The more people you tell, the more social pressure you'll feel to follow through and not back out at the last minute. Enter social networks. Nothing makes a better Facebook post than "I just signed up for my first fifty-miler!"

COACHING AND ULTRAMARATHONS

Runners sometimes hire coaches, and the practice is increasing. Years ago, many people assumed running was simple enough to be done without guidance. Personally, I blame this idea for the horrible running form we often see at road races.

A running coach can teach you a litany of useful skills, including good running form. A running coach can also set up a training plan, monitor your progress, and recommend changes to improve your performance. Coaches can also provide necessary encouragement and moral support.

Running coaches are relatively easy to find online. Simply Google "running coach [your municipality]." Running coaches in the United States are typically certified by Road Runners Club of America (RRCA) or United States Track and Field (USATF). I personally prefer the latter mostly because of my anti–road running bias. For trail running and ultramarathon coaching, definitely look for a coach that has actual hands-on experience.

KIDS AS ULTRARUNNERS

When I first started ultrarunning, a "young" ultrarunner was in his or her mid-twenties. Oh, how times have changed! Over the last year or two, a handful of kids under the age of fourteen have made news for running (and finishing) long ultras. To many, this is a shocking development for two reasons.

First, there are concerns for the kids' health. Specifically, what permanent damage may be done to their developing bodies? Ultras are hard on (snicker) our adult bodies; what effect will they have on the growth plates of bones, the endocrine system, etc.? This issue is legitimate. As of right now, there's no research on the effects of long-distance running on children's developing bodies. Jonathan Beverly of *Running Times* highlighted the lack of empirical evidence in his 2011 article titled "Should Kids Run Long?" His paraphrased conclusion: *with close monitoring, there's nothing wrong with children running long distances.*

Second, there are concerns for the kids' motives. Are they running long distances because they genuinely enjoy running long distances? Or are they running long distances because a parent or coach is pushing them? Over the years, I've spent a great deal of time around youth baseball, football, wrestling, MMA, soccer, basketball, and even running. It's obvious some parents overtly compel their kids to participate and it usually doesn't end well. These are the parents that mandate regular practices, cross-training, and focus on winning to the exclusion of anything and everything else. Sometimes parents drive their kids in more subtle ways, like showering the child with affection while they're participating. The result is a shift from intrinsic motivation (which is sustainable) to extrinsic motivation (which is not sustainable and eventually leads to burnout).

If your kid wants to run ultras, it's probably safe to allow him or her as long as him or her health is closely monitored. All the same rules apply. Make sure him or her getting a balanced diet, plenty of sleep, frequent rest days, and ease into training. Encourage him and her. If he or she begins experiencing burnout, let him or her stop.

BURNING RIVER PART II

About a week after I had finished the Hallucination 100, the soreness subsided enough for rosy recollection to set in. Maybe that race wasn't so hard after all. I decided to consider another hundred-miler. Two hours later, I was booking a hotel room in suburban Cleveland. I was going to avenge my 2008 DNF at Burning River!

I was positive I would be able to finish the race. Furthermore, I was sure I could do it *barefoot*. After all, I now knew what the entire one hundred miles felt like, and I was a much more experienced barefoot runner.

I continued training throughout that winter, which included some ridiculous barefoot runs in the snow. It seemed like a great way to help condition my body to the rigors of barefootedness in rough conditions. I even ran a variety of cold-weather road races barefoot that year, then eventually about fifty-four miles at the Mind the Ducks twelve-hour race in New York.

The obsession with barefoot running helped fuel my first foray into book writing. Since I was a professional educator, people seemed to naturally assume I could teach how to run barefoot. I organized a barefoot clinic, which had around fifteen attendees. I prepared a "how to run barefoot" binder for them, which was my very first nonacademic "writing project." Word spread, and a few other friends started requesting copies of the binder. Since it was heavy, the cost to ship it was somewhat prohibitive. I inquired about alternative formats at a local printing business. The owner suggested I have it bound as a paperback book. I spent a few days investigating things like layout and design, and half-jokingly told Shelly I should just write a book. Her response: "Why not?"

At that point, it didn't seem especially difficult. Most of the writing was done; I just needed to work out logistics like ISBN numbers (that number by the barcode) to sell the book via Amazon, editing, cover work, etc. I asked around and recruited a small army of fellow barefoot runners as my "production team." Within about two months, we managed to produce the very first copies of the first edition of *The Barefoot Running Book*.

The book itself was pretty bad. The writing was poor, there were no pictures or diagrams, and it was expensive due to the small printing quantities. As a testament to the laws of supply and demand, copies of this book occasionally pop up on eBay or Amazon for more than it cost to produce the original manuscript. Since it was the first "barefoot running" book to hit the market, I sold enough copies to eventually fund the expanded and significantly improved second edition. The second edition was eventually purchased by a publisher and updated to reflect my evolution of thoughts on barefoot and minimalist shoe running (hint: it's more about the form used than what you're wearing on your feet).

In 2008, there were very few runners trying to run trail hundred-milers barefoot. People like Leif Rustvold, Ted MacDonald, and Todd Ragsdale were attempting it, but none had succeeded. I saw it as a bit of a competition, and I wanted to win. Since I was familiar with the Burning River course, I was confident I'd be the first.

The preparation for BR part II went smoothly. My training was an extension of the previous year, though I swapped the weight lifting–heavy Crossfit workouts with more dynamic high intensity interval training with my friend Pete Kemme of kemmefitness.com. I continued weekly long runs, shorter fartlek runs, and hill repeats. I would occasionally hit the track and do 400- or 800-meter repeats. By early summer, I felt like I was fully prepared physically.

My intense, focused training was almost undone by an ill-timed stupid long run a month before Burning River. My friends Jesse Scott, Mark Robillard, and Jeremiah Cataldo decided to attempt a sixty-eight-mile training run on the Kal-Haven trail between Kalamazoo and South Haven, Michigan. It was a thirty-four-mile flat crushed limestone railroad-converted-to-trail route. We started around mid-afternoon so most of the run would take place in the dark. We were initially joined by elite barefoot runner James Webber, but he wisely turned around after a few miles.

We made it halfway.

We ran into multiple logistical problems, which forced us to abort the run at 1 a.m. . . . about three miles after we left Benton Harbor on the way back to the parking lot. We realized we had zero chance of getting everyone back to the car. We doubted we'd be able to make it back to South Haven and find an open business or use our one charged cell phone to call a relative. We were, after all, almost two hours away from home by car. We considered having the faster runners (Jesse and Jeremiah) run back to the car then pick Mark and me up, but the temperature was dropping faster than expected. It would take at least four or five hours for them to run the distance then drive back to us. With only thin, hot weather clothing, I was worried we'd be in danger of hypothermia. After brainstorming for a few minutes, we decided to try to call a taxi.

Luckily, we found one company that still had a driver on the road. We gave the dispatcher our location . . . which was an intersection of two rural roads in BFE. Naturally he was skeptical, so we had to explain the whole situation. There's something about verbalizing stupid running shenanigans to nonrunners that really highlights our ridiculousness.

The cab driver arrived about an hour later. After another hour ride, we arrived back at the trailhead parking lot. Broken and defeated, we took the natural course of action: breakfast at Denny's.

Jesse and I spent the next few days discussing the failed run. While we often appeared to be apathetic slackers, the failure stung. We *knew* we could do the double crossing, so we did the most logical thing. We decided to try again . . . four days after the first attempt. Mark was in, but Jeremiah (who was also running Burning River three weeks away) wisely declined. We recruited our friend Tony Schaub to ride a bike and serve as our "support vehicle." The food and water we had to carry the first time contributed to the failure. We also decided to start in the morning. The heat and humidity of the day would be easier to manage than the cold of the night.

The run went fairly well despite the thirty to forty miles we had run just four days earlier. It took somewhere around eighteen hours, which was a great opportunity to test all my gear and strategies for Burning River.

By the time the hundred-miler rolled around, most of the blisters and chafing had healed. I still felt some of the residual fatigue of the Kal-Haven run, but the inactivity between the runs served as an adequate taper. My crew for this time around consisted of Shelly, Jesse, and Andrew "Art" Brix, a barefoot running friend we knew from a running forum. We recruited Art mostly because a) he was willing, and b) he brewed his own unique beers.

The night before the race, the four of us were hanging out in our hotel room discussing race strategy. We were planning things such as pace, gear, and which crew member was going to pace me at various stages. We've always had a customary beer or three before a race, so we indulged in some of Art's beer.

It was good. *Too* good.

Around 1 a.m., one of us had a moment of clarity and realized the race started in four hours. When my alarm went off two and a half hours later, I was teetering in that weird stage between drunkedness and hangover. Luckily I had run enough races that my prerace routine didn't require much thought. I tried drinking as much water as possible to help limit the effects of the alcohol-induced dehydration, and managed to choke down a cream cheese muffin. Still, I was in rough shape.

The race started without much fanfare. The first few miles were terrible. It felt like I had been running for fifty miles. My vision was foggy and I was having trouble concentrating on the road (I was barefoot . . . this was supposed to be my chance to run the barefoot hundred-miler). I threw up once, then dry heaved every ten minutes or so. I was almost certain I would be forced to drop out of the race as soon as I saw my crew for the first time.

Luckily I didn't see my crew until around mile ten or so. I was beginning to feel a little better. I had instructed them to buy me a bacon, egg, and cheese biscuit meal from McDonald's (one of my favorite ultra foods). I drank the orange juice, choked down the hash browns, and took the sandwich with me as I headed out of the aid station. I took one bite and started to heave again. I tossed the remainder in the bushes. You know, to give the local raccoons a treat.

The water and Heed (my preferred sport drink) were helping to pull me out of my funk. By mile twenty I was actually feeling good. My feet held up well over the asphalt-covered first fifth of the course. The dehydration symptoms had subsided. I was riding a high. I was tempted to speed up a bit to make up for the time I lost dry heaving in the bushes but knew I had to reign myself in. There were still many miles ahead.

Around mile twenty-five, I hit an especially rough section of trails featuring large, sharp, unavoidable rocks. My feet took

201

a beating. By the time I hit the crushed limestone tow path trail a few miles before the mile thirty-three aid station, I was ready to abandon the barefoot idea. If I continued, I knew I wouldn't make it to the halfway point. When I entered the aid station, I asked for the "emergency huaraches" I had packed just in case. I was so confident in my barefoot prowess I hadn't packed any other shoes. The huaraches were in one of my bags the crew had left in the car, so Jesse took off to find them.

I was relaxing, drinking some soda, and eating some food. I had cleaned off my feet and slipped on my Injinji toe socks. About ten minutes later, Jesse breathlessly returned without the huaraches. He couldn't find them. I was annoyed, but tried not to get too upset. Shelly suddenly remembered there were two bags in the car, so Jesse took off again. About ten minutes later, he returned with an entire gear bag. He didn't want to take the time to dig through it, so he brought the whole thing. I was now having difficulty containing my anger; I had wasted close to thirty minutes in the aid station. I slipped on the huaraches and headed out.

The trail ran along a road lined with cars of the various runners' crews. About twelve minutes after leaving the aid station, I came upon our car. I looked down at my Garmin. It was exactly one mile from the aid station. I suddenly felt really bad for acting angry because Jesse took so long—he had just run four five-minute miles, the last of which carrying a huge gear bag over his head. I learned an important lesson: *never get angry at your crew.*

I would live by that code for about one year . . . until the "battery incident" in the middle of the night during the Western States hundred-miler.

The huaraches, despite having only a six millimeter thick sole, helped immensely. They provided just enough protection to keep a good pace. The only other noteworthy event happened around mile forty. I was absentmindedly jogging along when I felt a sudden intense, sharp stabbing pain at the base of my right Achilles tendon. I had learned enough about anatomy via barefoot running to know what probably just happened—my Achilles just separated from my ankle. I stopped running and panicked for exactly two seconds until another sudden sharp stabbing pain struck my left thigh. Then I heard the buzzing.

Fucking angry bees!

I took off sprinting for a half mile. When I no longer heard the buzzing, I stopped. The pain in my ankle and thigh wasn't really subsiding. Upon closer inspection, the stingers were still embedded. I scraped them out with my fingernails. As I was doing this, I realized just how lucky I had been. I forgot to mention a small detail: I was running in a kilt, and was going commando. The bee that stung my thigh was dangerously close to my junk. That would be the second-to-the-last time I ever raced in a kilt. I'm a slow learner.

The rest of the race was pretty standard for a hundred-miler. Eventually I picked up Shelly as a pacer, then switched off to Jesse for the night. By that time, I was in pretty rough shape. We more or less walked through the entire night. I picked up Shelly with two sections to go. The first was ridiculously slow as I continued to mostly walk. When we got to the last aid station, Shelly changed up her strategy. She convinced me to run to a traffic cone about 150 yards ahead. I complied, though I was running like Frankenstein. After a short walk break, she did it again. Running felt a little better. Sensing I had some running left in me, Shelly told me our friend Jimmy Viggiano, who was running his first hundred-miler, was right behind me. My competitive streak kicked in and I started running without breaks.

My pace slowly crept lower and lower, from thirteen-minute miles to twelve, then down to eleven. I started passing a few runners. I got down to about ten-minute miles. With about a mile left, I flirted with a nine-minute pace. By the time I crossed the finish line, I had averaged a respectable twelve-minute pace for the entire section. After receiving my buckle, I think I may have stumbled off to the side, collapsed, and immediately fell asleep.

Avenging the previous DNF was sweet, but the real breakthrough occurred because I had managed to overcome the stupid long run a few weeks earlier, survived the hangover, and managed to run hard at the very end of the race. I was learning more and more about my capabilities, which would fuel future training and race strategy. Perhaps most importantly, I made the decision to abandon the goal of running a hundred-miler barefoot. Actually improving at ultras was a more important goal.

Two weeks after Burning River, I decided to run a local trail marathon. It absolutely sucked. I was physically wrecked from the Kal-Haven run and Burning River. I learned another valuable lesson: recovery is as important as training. The situation was made worse by the fact that I had decided to run barefoot and wear the kilt one last time. The unavoidable rocks and twigs that littered the course took a toll on my feet. When I got to the last aid station, I sat down and elevated my battered bare feet on another chair. One of the volunteers shook his head and said "I can clearly see you're nuts." To this day, I'm not sure if that was a bare feet or kilt reference. Bad puns are a staple for aid station volunteers.

SECTION 6:
PLANNING FOR ULTRAMARATHONS

FINDING THE TIME TO TRAIN FOR ULTRAS

Ultramarathons must take a ton of training. Don't they?

That's a question I receive more than any other. Well, aside from "Why do you do it?" People are hesitant to make the plunge into the world of ultras because the training appears so intimidating. It must take a gargantuan weekly time commitment to prepare your body to run over thirty-one miles at one time.

Yes and no.

It is possible to run an ultra on very little training. As I mentioned earlier, my friend Rich Elliott decided to run a marathon and then a fifty-miler with no training. His lone training run consisted of a 5k a few weeks prior to the longer race. That's it. He ran 3.1 training miles in two years. On race day of the fifty, he managed to eek out twenty-seven miles before throwing in the towel.

John DeVries, another good friend and the Crossfit trainer that helped me prepare for one of my hundred-milers, ran a twelve-hour timed ultra with a single eight-mile run in the previous two years. He made it to about twenty-two miles.

What can be learned from their experiences? It's tough to run an ultra with no training. If you have a little bit of a running background, you could probably do it with minimal training. If you have a strong running background, you can probably do it with the training you already have.

The correlation should be obvious: *the more you train, the better the results*. I would go a step further and say the more you train, the *more enjoyable the race will be*.

It does take time. This *is* a huge undertaking, and you *will* have to work to do it. There are no substitutes or shortcuts—you have to put in the hours. It's not like triathlons where you can drop a grand on aerodynamic berets or fancy "lighter-than-farts" bolts to save a few ounces . . . you gotta bust your ass!

However, these hours don't have to be intimidating. You don't have to add a ton of training hours on top of your already busy schedule. The trick is to merge your ultra training with your existing daily life.

Not only is it possible, it's the norm. Ultrarunning is a unique sport. Even the best of the best don't make enough money from sponsorships or race winnings to make a living. In fact, this money rarely pays for the races themselves. Pretty much all ultra-runners have normal jobs. They have to figure out how to fit ultrarunning into their lives.

The secret is deceptively simple:

Always Train

No, I don't mean skirt all your responsibilities, sell the kids on eBay, and start running ten hours each day. Look at everything you do on a daily basis and begin asking: *How can I tweak this activity to achieve some training benefit?*

Turn everything in your life into an opportunity to train. By simply reframing the situation, you don't have to worry about carving four hours each day from your already busy life. Instead you are now free to train twenty-four hours a day, seven days a week! Day at the office? Training. Picking up toilet bowl cleaner from the grocery store? Training. Puttin' the moves on your significant other? Training. Yes, you read that right. Sounds more fun than running around a track, huh?

BALANCING LIFE COMMITMENTS

Training for ultras takes significant time, even if you go to great lengths to incorporate training in every element of your daily life. Managing your family and/or professional life can be a challenge. If you don't have a spouse, kids, or even a job, congratulations! You've met all the qualifications for becoming a professional ultrarunner! Enjoy that ride as long as you can. You'll never have this much free time again. Well, at least not for a number of decades.

In the event you do have a spouse, kids, and/or a career, balancing these responsibilities can be a challenge. Here's some practical advice:

- **Set priorities.** Mine always went something like this: time with spouse, time with kids, ultra training, catching up on my favorite TV shows, work-related stuff, chores, grooming facial hair.

- **Develop a training schedule that has a minimal impact on other responsibilities.** This may involve training after everyone else goes to bed or before they wake up in the morning.
- **If you have to miss a workout, don't fret.** Missing a single workout isn't going to doom your plan.
- **Give your spouse plenty of time to follow his or her own hobbies.** We all need our own "me" time. It may also help to lavish his or her with gifts.
- **Understand that most opposition to an ultrarunning spouse is rooted in resentment.** The non-running spouse feels as if his or her shouldering an unfair burden. Having open, honest communication about sharing responsibilities will usually cure this issue.
- **Bring your kids with you using a jogging stroller or, if they're old enough, have them ride their bikes behind you.** Better yet, have them man an aid station for you.
- **Get your spouse hooked on running ultras, too.** It's better to fight over who gets to train than having to defend the need to train. And the endorphines and dopamine will probably enhance your sex life. Win-win.

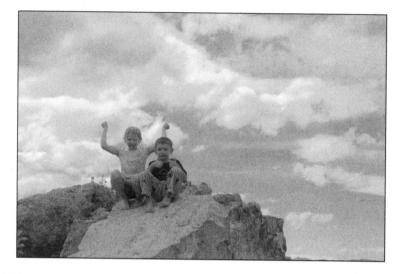

When I was building my endurance base early in my ultrarunning days, Shelly and I were having lots of babies. When the babies got on a fairly reliable sleep schedule, I'd leave to run after they woke up in the middle of the night. I would tend to their needs, then put them back to sleep. Once they were sleeping, I'd run. This allowed Shelly to sleep for a few hours undisturbed and allowed me to stick to my training plan. As our kids aged, finding time to train became easier.

IS THERE SUCH THING AS A PERFECT CAREER FOR ULTRAMARATHONERS?

When I talked about the idea of thinking of every moment of your life as an opportunity to train, I bet you started considering your profession. I did the same thing. I used to be a high school teacher. When I started running ultras, I looked for every opportunity I could find to train.

It started with parking as far away from the front doors as possible, which forced me to walk farther. If I had to go anywhere around the school and time wasn't an issue, I took a route that would bring me up and down multiple sets of stairs. Sometimes I would eat a huge lunch; sometimes I would fast . When teaching, I'd stand on a balance board to build balance and core strength. I would even do some air squats and walking lunges at the beginning and end of every day to help develop leg strength.

I've had a variety of jobs that provided excellent ultra training. I've worked as a seasonal "driver's helper" for UPS during the holiday season, which involved carrying boxes from the car (what they call their trucks) to doorsteps. This often involved stairs. Being a training dork, I wore my Garmin GPS watch for a week. On an average day, I would hastily walk anywhere between seven to ten miles and climb and descend around six thousand stairs. I also worked in a lumberyard where I assisted customers in loading their purchases. This included cinder blocks, two by fours, ninety pound bags of concrete, and even twelve by twelve by twenty foot beams. I would walk anywhere between two and four miles each day and lift ridiculously heavy shit all day long. Both jobs were so intense, I didn't have to do any supplemental training.

There are some other careers that can offer even more opportunities to train. Anyone who spends time on their feet can think of that as a form of training. Lift heavy objects? That builds strength. Work in a skyscraper? What better way to develop hill climbing and descending ability than avoiding the elevator. Exotic dancer? Pole dancing is perhaps the best core-building exercise out there.

If you are interested in ultras and happen to be looking for a career, consider the training prospects. Something like a walking mail delivery route could make for wonderful training. Better yet, how about working as a mountain guide? Working in an office? Look for a place that will allow a stand-up desk. Better yet, how about a treadmill desk? If you're not fortunate enough to be in the market for a new career, look at your present career. Make a game out of finding new and interesting training opportunities.

This is also a good opportunity for me to toss in one of my major life philosophies—*work to live, don't live to work.* Shelly and I both take jobs that we not only enjoy but also allow us to have ample free time. We work enough to pay the bills, do the things we truly enjoy, and tuck a little away for future expenses (kids' college, retirement, rainy day fund, etc.). We save money by not wasting income on things that aren't important to us and avoid debt whenever possible. This strategy has allowed us to travel frequently, spend lots of time with our children, engage in creative endeavors, and pursue our hobbies in earnest.

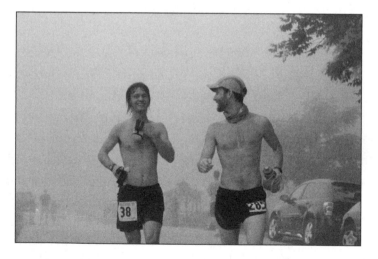

Ben VanHoose and Jeremiah Cataldo.

HOW DO YOU CHOOSE A TRAINING PLAN?

Okay, let's get down to the nitty-gritty of ultra training: the plan. The training plan is the backbone of your quest to finish your first ultra. If you do a quick Internet search, you'll find dozens of plans dedicated specifically to ultras. On top of that, you'll also find hundreds of marathon training plans that feasibly could be modified for ultras.

You probably want me to recommend one specific plan, huh?

Too bad. I'm going to make *you* choose. I'll give you some guidance, but ultimately the decision has to be yours to make.

I presented a few of the more popular plans above. The following is the criteria I recommend to make the choice. You should be able to quickly peruse the details of each plan and get an idea of those that might work well for you.

Let's start with the criteria. These should be your primary considerations:

- **Consideration #1: What distance am I running?** Some plans are specifically tailored to a given distance. Others can be modified for any distance. You can start by eliminating those which cannot be modified to fit your given distance.

- **Consideration #2: How does the schedule of training runs (and cross-training in some cases) fit your life?** If you work eighty hours a week, a plan that requires several long, slow runs each week probably won't work. Make sure the plan fits your time allotment. And stop pissing away your life by working too much.

- **Consideration #3: Does this running plan have a community I can lean on for support?** Some plans (like Crossfit Endurance) have an active community of people going through the exact same thing you are. It can be handy to lean on them for support and guidance as you progress toward the race.

THE INHERENT PROBLEMS WITH FOLLOWING ELITE TRAINING PLANS OR RESEARCH

When I start offering advice for training plans, many people invariably ignore the "experimentation" idea and request a training routine "proven" by research or request a plan used by elite runners. Both approaches have similar fundamental flaws.

First, we're all individuals with unique physical and mental capacities. Research is usually conducted on a small sample of athletes, thus cannot be effectively generalized. A good example are Tabata intervals. In 1996, Dr. Izimi Tabata and his research team published a study showing how a particular workout routine ("Tabatas") increased the VO2 max of speed skaters. The fitness industry immediately adopted the workout and started using it for any and all purposes. Personally, I like Tabata intervals because they're fun. However, they're not a magic pill. They are not necessarily going to make or break you as an ultrarunner.

Second, elites usually have a long history of building athleticism. Many elite ultrarunners have a history of competitive running (track and field, cross country, etc.). They've spent the majority of their lives training. A random inactive person following their exact same routine isn't going to produce the same results because they don't have the years and years of relevant experience.

Third, we rarely get a full picture of an elite's training regimen. We don't see their diet. We don't see their sleep patterns. We don't see their sports massage sessions. We don't see their frequency of sexual activity (surely they're getting lots of action; ultrarunners are known for their hordes of sex-crazed groupies). We don't see their periodization (do they have an "off season"?) All of these elements play into the success elites have. This same argument can be used for research participants. While experimenters may attempt to control all extraneous variables and use statistics to assess the generalizability of any given study, the results still may not apply to you.

Fourth, elites and their training may not necessarily follow known best practices. Granted, "known best practices" is pretty vague and open to interpretation, but it's never safe to assume everything elite runners do leads to better performance. It's not uncommon to hear stories of elite ultrarunners chugging diet soda or eating a steady diet of fast food. Would this work for all of us? Probably not.

Fifth, some self-described "experts" really aren't that good. I met a man at a clinic that was devoutly religious. He read the Bible daily and claimed he got all of his training advice from John 3:16. Naturally I was skeptical; this John fellow's 3:16 wouldn't even qualify for Boston.

GIVE ME A TRAINING PLAN!

Here are a few popular training plans for the new ultrarunner. This isn't meant to be an exhaustive list but rather a few examples to give you a taste of what's out there. I've used a few and will give my own comments when appropriate.

- **Crossfit/Crossfit Endurance**: Crossfit is a functional fitness-based workout program designed to develop multiple areas of athletic skills. CF *Endurance* adds an element of high-intensity anaerobic running to the mix. The theory goes something like this: By running long, slow distances, we get slower and weaker. If we do shorter distance high-intensity running combined with functional fitness training, we get faster and stronger at running (and any other athletic endeavor). I've used CF/CFE in the past, and still use many elements of the program. It's good. However, the lack of long runs severely dampens the ability to experiment with all of the variables inherent in ultras (like gear, food, chafing, etc.). If you like your workouts to end with lying in the fetal position in a pool of your own vomit, this is the plan for you.

- **Maffetone Method**: The Maffetone Method pretty much takes the opposite approach. It replaces all high-intensity workouts with long, slow runs. The Maffetone method uses a heart rate monitor to keep heart rate below a predetermined point to train your body to utilize fat burning. Higher-intensity workouts can be added after an endurance base has been built. I have played around with the Maffetone heart rate monitoring, and it does work as advertised. If you don't like sweating, this is the plan for you.

- **Modified Hal Higdon plan**: Hal Higdon's marathon training programs have been guiding marathoners to the finish line for . . . well, forever. His plans have a balance of different types of runs based on experience. The tricky part? His plans are designed for marathons. They can be modified easily, though. If you like doing what everybody else is doing, this is the plan for you.

- **Jeff Galloway–based plan**: Galloway's plans, like Higdon's, are designed for marathons. However, Galloway's plan differs by utilizing a system of running and walking intervals. This concept is one of the most popular techniques used in ultras. As such, his training plan is quite popular. So popular in fact, ultrarunner Tim Looney refers to ultras as giant "Gallo-walking festivals." If you spend your mornings doing laps at the local mall and watching *The Golden Girls* because of all the hotties, this is the plan for you.

- ***Runner's World* plan**: *Runner's World* produced an ultra training plan, but it assumes you've already run a marathon. Still, some people like *Runner's World*. Their forums are pretty cool. And some people like the incredible diversity of their magazine's cover art. You know, a skinny white girl with ash blonde hair one month, then a skinny white girl with strawberry blonde hair the next. Anyway, here's the plan: *www.runnersworld.com/article/0,7120,s6-238-244--7556-0,00.html.*

- **Santa Clara Runners customizable plan**: This plan is really cool—it's an interactive website that produces a customized plan. The plan itself is basic; there are no specifications for different types of runs. Still, it will get you to the finish line. Check it out here: *www.scrunners. org/ultrasch.php.*

- **The plan from *The Barefoot Running Book***: I wrote a plan included in my other book, but it's designed for marathons. Same deal as Higdon's and Galloway's plans… it can be modified for ultras. It's really a hybrid that combines Crossfit and Crossfit-style workouts designed in conjunction with my friend Pete Kemme of Kemme Fitness (*http://kemmefitness.com*) and Maffetone's long, slow runs. It's the best of both worlds!

- ***Relentless Forward Progress* plan**: Bryon Powell's excellent book *Relentless Forward Progress* includes an excellent plan based on Bryon's own experiences. Bryon is the editor-in-chief of irunfar.com, *the* ultramarathon news resource on the web. If you're looking for a more legitimate, serious book by ultrarunners that are actually *talented, hard-working runners*, check out his book.

Each one of these plans takes a different approach to training. Using the criteria I shared earlier, pick the plan that will be a good fit for you. If you can't decide, pick the plan from *The Barefoot Running Book*. If you are offended by my shameless cross-promotion, pick Crossfit. Then send me the pictures of you lying in that pool of vomit.

DO YOU HAVE TO FOLLOW THE PLAN RELIGIOUSLY?

Now that you have a plan, the next question revolves around adaptability. Do you have to follow the plan precisely?

It probably depends on who you ask.

Those with a type A personality will insist you follow the workout precisely. If you miss a run, the world will come crashing down. It's a moot point, though, because your run should be at the top of your list of the other 498 things you have to do each day.

As you probably guessed, I'm not really a list-making kind of person. I'm more of a realist. I'm also guessing you're not really a type A personality, either. After all, you *are* reading a book of questionable quality with a ridiculous title written by a mediocre runner.

If you miss a run, it's not a big deal. In fact, taking a break occasionally gives your body time to heal. If you do miss a workout, just move on to the next one.

PERIODIZATION

Periodization is a process of preparing for ultras by building specific skills at specific times. It usually begins with an endurance base–building phase, followed by a hill climbing and descending phase (or strength training), followed by a speed-building phase.

The idea works fairly well. By introducing each concept separately, you can develop each skill faster than if you were to do all three simultaneously. You begin with the most general skills (running long distances). As your goal race nears, you hone the specific skills needed for the ultra.

I used a system of periodization for my first ultra. I spent twelve weeks building my endurance base, six weeks working on speed, and six weeks working on specific trails. Note that I didn't do any hill training. It was a huge mistake. The hills on the course absolutely killed me. Live and learn.

PLAN AN OFF-SEASON

When I first started dabbling in ultrarunning, I was lucky to have a naturally occurring off-season in the form of winter. The bitter cold, wind, snow, and lack of motivation due to seasonal affective disorder combined to give me a solid two or three months of minimal running. I did some running during this time to maintain an endurance base, but the overall training volume decreased by at least 75 percent. This off-season allowed my body to heal from the rigors of the previous year. It also helped ward off burnout. By the time the warmth of spring arrived, I was ready to get back to heavy training. When scheduling races and designing a training plan, take at least four to six weeks off at some point during the year. Your short-term fitness may take a small hit, but your long-term fitness will prosper.

RACE STRATEGY

How do you plan for a race measured in hours? I will sometimes overhear runners discussing 5k strategy. It usually involves running at a specified intensity for various intervals with the goal of finishing as quickly as possible. Personally, I've always used a "run as fast as you can" strategy . . . which may explain why I suck at 5ks. Anyway, I digress.

Needless to say, ultramarathons require a different strategy than the faster, shorter races. Even a typical marathon strategy won't necessarily be effective. Important note: I'm assuming you are not planning on winning the ultra; your goal is to finish. Lazy runners don't plan to win.

Before we delve into detail, there are a few universal differences between ultras and subultras. The longer the ultra, the greater this difference.

- Walking is acceptable. Only the elites will run the entire time.
- Eating *during* the run is more or less required.

- Ultras are about surviving . . . you always have to assess the cumulative effects of your decisions. A bad decision early in a race will haunt you throughout.

Okay, now we tackle strategy.

The first thing to consider: The distance. Generally speaking, longer races require more walking. In a fifty-mile race, you may walk a total of ten miles. In a hundred-mile race, you may walk thirty to fifty miles.

The second consideration: Cutoff times. Most races will set an absolute time before everyone packs up and goes home. Most races will require you to meet certain time checkpoints. If you fall behind these checkpoints, you will be removed from the race.

The third consideration: Terrain. A flat course will require a much different strategy than a mountainous course. When assessing terrain, it is also useful to note the different obstacles you will encounter. Will the course consist of asphalt? Dirt trails? Sand? Lots of rocks and/or roots (technical trail?) Stairs? Steep hills? It is easier to run faster on certain surfaces; this will play a role in planning.

The fourth consideration: Fitness. The greater your fitness level, the faster and longer you will be able to run. Personally, I usually overestimate my fitness level. I am slowly learning how my body will react to long distances, which results in a better plan.

The fifth consideration: Aid stations. The time does not stop while you're gorging yourself on M&Ms and salted potatoes. The time spent in aid stations will affect your overall finish time.

As such, it is necessary to factor this into planning. I like to plan on a five-minute stop at each aid station. I tell my crew to keep the stops under one minute. Depending on how much primping I need, my time usually falls between those two times.

The sixth consideration: Slowing as the race progresses. Remember, you're a lazy runner. You won't be running negative splits in an ultra. Assume your second-half pace will be significantly slower than the first-half pace.

The seventh consideration: Weather. Some conditions, such as heavy rain (and subsequent mud), snow, high heat, oppressive humidity, or strong winds can slow you down. It is important to estimate the climate and local weather before developing a race strategy.

The last consideration: Strategy. Now that you have done the requisite research, you will be prepared to map out a strategy. How exactly you devise that plan will depend on your organizational habits. I like to estimate a variety of finish times with the elapsed time I would expect to reach each aid station. Once the calculations are made, I print a chart. If weather is expected to be wet, I laminate it. It takes some work, but it gives me an easy-to-follow spreadsheet that I can use during the race to determine if I am going too slow or too fast.

Warning: *Make sure your crew understands your chart.* Luckily, my first hundred-mile finish was helped significantly by Michael Helton's ability to interpret my laminated poster board–sized spreadsheet filled with mileage numbers and times. Michael deciphered this between rushing from one aid station to the next. It would have been wise to explain my system *before* the race started.

I find it is easier if I don't plan specific times for walk breaks. In my first hundred-mile attempt, I had planned every single walk break throughout the race. Not only was it incredibly time-consuming but it was impossible to follow once the race started. It served as a major distraction. Some runners will use a specific time ratio to determine walking breaks. I have experimented with this idea extensively and was never able to find a good solution that worked well. Now I use more of a Zen-like approach and walk when I feel like it.

The race strategy you map out will go a long way toward preventing the unexpected. Still, the more potential problems you can anticipate, the greater the likelihood of finishing.

Overplanning can be dangerous, too. You cannot predict every single issue that may arise. Some problems require you to fix them as they arise. Experience will improve those problem-solving abilities, as will long training runs.

AID STATIONS AND STRATEGY

Aid stations are one of my favorite elements of ultras. At worst, they are a candy and snack food–filled oasis in the middle of the wilderness that offer a quick break from the monotony of slugging along the trail. At best, they're a roaring party where everyone is singing, dancing, and drinking and you're treated as the guest of honor.

A typical aid station will stock sweet carbohydrate-rich foods, salty snacks, fruit, sandwiches, water, and one or two sports drinks. They will also carry basic supplies like adhesive bandages, insect repellent, sunscreen, and petroleum jelly. Well-stocked aid stations may also cook a variety of hot food, coffee, or even pizza. Some aid stations may also have medical personnel on hand.

Aid stations are almost exclusively staffed by volunteers. Sometimes the volunteers will be veteran ultrarunners that have seen it all. These volunteers are an invaluable resource as they can provide expert advice. You have a problem? They know how to fix it. Other times the volunteers may be ultra rookies and this is their first exposure to the sport. In either case, treat each volunteer with respect. They're donating their time for your benefit. Never yell or swear at a volunteer; always say please and thank you.

Before running an ultra, it's important to consider and practice aid station strategies. Time spent at aid stations is time wasted by not moving forward. At the 2008 Burning River 100, I planned on spending no more than thirty seconds at each aid station. At that point, I had only run two fifty-milers and hadn't developed (or practiced) a good aid station routine. In the rush to keep moving, I missed some important details . . . like forgetting to eat. The problem was compounded because I hadn't thoroughly explained the role my crew would play. As the race wore on and problems mounted, we wasted a lot of time digging through my excessive gear. I spent more and more time at aid stations. That, coupled with my inadequate training and lack of mental toughness, resulted in a DNF.

In later ultras, I learned how to prepare myself and crew for aid stations. If I had a multiple-member crew, I gave each one tasks. I developed an efficient routine. I closely monitored time. Eventually my aid station strategy became a competitive advantage instead of a liability.

So how should you go about preparing for aid stations? Practice is the key. I actually set up a small folding table in my yard, stocked it with some supplies, and practiced my routine. It would start as I approached the table. I would decide exactly what I needed to do based on the mental checklist of the problems I needed to fix. I would drink anything remaining in my water bottle(s) and unscrew the top, consolidate any garbage to a single pocket, and if I needed to replace flashlight batteries, I'd shut it off and unscrew the top. Once I arrived at the table, I'd put the plan in action. If there were volunteers, I'd give them the bottle to refill, deposit trash, and replace the batteries. I would then eat whatever I could from the table while changing any clothing that needed changing. Next would be foot care if needed, which usually involved sitting. I would then get more food, then relube anything that was in danger of chafing. I would make one last stop at the table, eat electrolytes if needed, fill my pockets with gels, take a drink, and grab my filled bottle(s) and one piece of wrapperless (no littering that way) food for the trail. Without a crew, I could get out of the aid station in about one minute depending on the attention my feet required. With my experienced crew members, I could do all of this in roughly thirty to forty seconds.

The key is practice. Aid stations, especially in your first few races, can be hectic. Practice gives you the confidence to calmly and methodically accomplish all that needs to be done. If you plan on using a crew (and/or pacers), it's useful to have them go through a few aid station practice sessions. The less ultra experience your crew has, the more important the practice becomes.

It's also useful to eliminate any germophobe tendencies before experiencing aid stations. Almost all of the food is communal. Lots of sweaty hands will be molesting that bowl of candy corn. Thinking about where those hands have been over the last forty-six miles would be like illuminating a hotel room with a black light—do your best to avoid it.

DROP BAGS

What is a drop bag?

A drop bag is some sort of container used to hold supplies needed during a race. The drop bag is dropped at some point along the race route. You will have access to the bag when you reach that part of the course.

Is a drop bag actually a bag?

Not necessarily, though that is the most common container. Some people use backpacks, duffel bags, plastic shopping bags, or garbage bags. Other containers can be used, too. I like Rubbermaid containers. Some people use five-gallon buckets. More or less any container will work, though it should be watertight. Each race may have specific rules that dictate size, shape, and acceptable containers.

Do you need drop bags?

If you have a crew and that crew has access to every aid station where drop bags are allowed, then no. If your crew does not have access to some drop bag locations, they can be useful.

What goes in the drop bags?

Drop bags can be used to stash almost any supplies needed for the race. Common contents include things like food, gels (technically food . . . but barely), electrolytes, first aid crap, lube, dry socks, spare clothes, rain gear, sunscreen, insect repellent, antidiarrhea meds, batteries, or whatever else you think you need. Maybe toss in a vibrator for a little "middle-of-the-race-natural-pain-relief" session?

How do you know if you pack too much?

For my first ultra, I had about twelve five-quart Rubbermaid containers full of assorted "goodies." Each drop "bag" was packed with everything I thought I would need. That turned out to be a huge mistake. When I arrived at the aid station, it took way too long to dig through the container to find what I needed. I had a ton of crap that just got in the way.

So how do you determine what is needed? Make a list of everything you think you need. Figure out what items will be available at the aid station and remove them from your list. Now eliminate unnecessary items (no need for batteries at an aid station you'll pass at noon). Now put everything else in the drop bag. Go to an open field and throw it as far as you can. If you can't throw it more than twenty feet, you packed too much.

PACERS

A pacer is a runner that runs with you during an ultramarathon. In most cases, pacers are allowed to join you in the later stages of a race. While many shorter ultras allow pacers, they're most commonly found in hundred-milers or longer.

A pacer serves as a guide, motivator, coach, entertainer, and cheerleader. A pacer does so much more than simply set the running pace. A good pacer keeps you on the course. He or she reminds you to eat and drink. He or she helps you survive the lows and ride the highs. When the shit hits the fan and things go south, your pacer is there to problem solve to get you to the finish line.

I've been fortunate to have a string of incredible pacers over the years. At the 2012 Grindstone 100, Shelly paced me for the last thirty-three miles. While I didn't experience a serious low, there were a few times I was discouraged about the slow pace needed to climb the rocky mountain trails. She kept me distracted, reminded me to eat, and monitored my well-being. When we finally hit a runnable section, she encouraged me to run. When we hit the last ten miles and I was fighting serious sleep deprivation, she took the lead on the trails to guide me through the rock fields.

I've had other great pacers, too. I credit my finish at Western States last year to Jeremiah Cataldo and Shelly. Jeremiah somehow managed to push me through thirty-plus miles in the darkness to put me in a position for a sub-twenty-four hour finish, then Shelly closed the deal over the last eight miles.

Prior to that, I've been paced by Jesse Scott, Mark Robillard, Michael Helton, and Stuart Peterson . . . all did fantastic jobs of leading me to my first two hundred-miler finishes. The value of a good pacer cannot be understated.

What Makes a Good Pacer?

It's tough to nail down exactly what qualities exemplify a great pacer because all runners will have slightly different needs. A good pacer should be able to adapt his or her strategies to maximize his or her runner's potential. Here are some considerations:

- **Pacing:** If the runner has a time goal, the pacer should try to set a pace that will reach said goal. The pacer should also be aware of contingency plans if that time goal is unattainable. Pushing too hard too early will usually result in a serious crash, which may lead the runner to drop from the race (DNF). The pacer has to be conservative, but not *too* conservative.
- **Position:** Does the runner prefer to lead or follow the pacer? Both positions have advantages and disadvantages. A pacer in the lead can look for course markings. A pacer that follows can closely monitor his or her runner. Since most predatory animals attack from behind, a dedicated

pacer that chose to follow could really take one for the team. I usually prefer to lead unless I need to speed up or I'm crossing technical terrain and have trouble seeing the trail (like at night when really tired). Watching the pacer's foot placement makes it easier to navigate the technical stuff.

- **Problem prevention:** A good pacer will recognize when the runner is about to have a problem. Did the runner suddenly get quiet? Maybe he or she is about to bonk (physical and psychological low caused by glycogen depletion). Did his or her running gait suddenly change? He or she may be developing a blister or other injury. Is he or she shivering or sweating profusely? He or she is too cold or too hot. Is he or she suddenly farting up a storm? he or she is having gastrointestinal distress. There are a thousand possible issues that can arise, and a good pacer will be able to recognize many of them *before* they become serious issues. I've been fortunate to have experienced ultrarunners (Shelly, Jeremiah, and Jesse) as pacers for the vast majority of my paced races. I regularly run with all three, so they know me well. They can predict problems a little earlier than someone that's not familiar with my idiosyncrasies.

- **Problem solving:** Okay, so the pacer doesn't *always* catch problems before they become problems. If things *do* go bad, the pacer is the runner's first line of defense to right the ship. This gets a little complicated because pacers can't "mule" (carry any gear for the runner), so the pacer can only work with whatever the runner is carrying. The pacer may have to force the runner to eat, drink, speed up, sit down to rest, sleep briefly along the trail, hold his or her hair if he or she is puking, pop blisters, lube unsavory parts of his or her body . . . whatever. It's important for the pacer to know *how* to solve any problem that arises. This is why experienced ultrarunners usually make the best pacers. Alternatively, novice pacers should be well-read on the issues facing ultrarunners.

- **Develop thick skin:** I like to think I'm a fairly even-keeled ultrarunner. . . . I try not to get too upset with my crew or pacers. However, running for twelve-plus hours tends to expose some raw nerves. A pacer should be ready for crabbiness and whining from his or her runner . . . and be ready to respond accordingly.

- **Physical durability:** Pacing is demanding. Depending on how long the pacer will be pacing, the pacer may go through many of the same experiences as the runner. He or she is going to get sleepy, fatigued, experience some pain, get hot or cold, experience lows . . . whatever. If pacers do experience anything negative, they have to shut the fuck up and keep it to themselves. Pacers can't complain. Pacers can't focus on themselves. Pacers can't quit because *they're* experiencing trouble.

- **Knowing when to quit:** Most new ultrarunners take an "I'm going to finish no matter what" strategy, which works great in theory. In reality, it's unlikely most people have experienced the cornucopia of shittiness that can occur late in an ultra. I've met very few people that seem to have the ability to keep plugging along *no matter what* (Ryan Hansard and Katie Zopf, I'm talking about you).

Everyone else will talk themselves into quitting at some point. A good pacer knows how to keep his or her runner going. He or she also knows when it's best to throw in the towel and fight another day.

- **Experience or familiarity?** My friend Vanessa asked if it's better to have a pacer that's an experienced ultrarunner that *doesn't* know you well or a newbie ultrarunner that *does* know you well. There are pros and cons to each. If you *have* to choose, experience is probably a safer bet. If someone has run quite a few ultras, He or she will know a variety of solutions to common problems. You know he or she has the tenacity to actually run the distances pacing requires. Conversely, a newbie may know you well, but won't know how to fix unexpected problems that arise. Either way, both trump inexperienced strangers. Most people like to think they have what it takes to run ultras, and they're probably right. Pacing isn't a very good proving ground, however.

Learning to Become a Pacer

Learning to pace is pretty straight forward. Do research and gain experience. The best places to gain research are ultra books like Bryon Powell's *Relentless Forward Progress* or Kevin Sayers's "Ultrunr" website. To gain experience, volunteer to work an aid station at the later stages of any ultramarathon. Volunteer to work as a crew member for someone running an ultra. Run an ultra yourself. Pay attention to other runners, pacers, and crew members. Be a sponge and absorb as much as you possibly can.

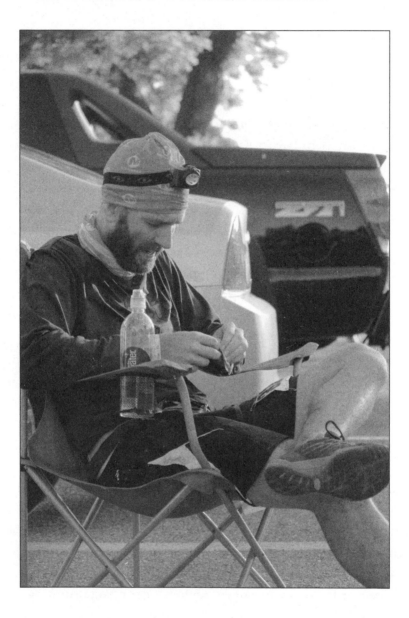

CREW

A crew is a person or group of people that help an ultramarathon runner complete the race by providing support along the course. The crew is sometimes known as "handlers," but I think the term is dorky. "Crew" sounds more like an entourage. I'm not hitting the night clubs with my "handlers."

The crew will follow the runner from location to location. Most races have specific locations where a crew can meet its runner, which is almost always at specific aid stations. These aid stations are said to allow "crew access." Depending on the rules of the particular race, crew access is usually explicitly limited to the aid station itself. The crew can't help the runner along the course or even a few hundred meters before or after the aid station.

The experience of crewing is defined by long periods of waiting, followed by a minute or two of frantic activity, followed by driving to the next location and repeating the cycle.

The crew's responsibilities are somewhat similar to a pit crew in auto racing. Since the runner wants to waste as little time as possible at each stop, the crew must quickly identify and correct any problems. They fill water bottles, suggest appropriate foods, and squeegee the sweat off your back. The crew must also keep the runner updated with information like his or her position relative to the cutoff times, place in the race (if the runner cares), any significant weather changes, or other pertinent information.

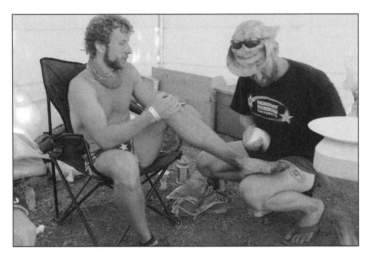

Crewing for Jesse Scott at Tahoe Rim, 2012.

The crew also has to be self-sufficient. The members have to be familiar with the course and race rules, know how to navigate from one crew access point to the next, and be prepared for the long hours of waiting. Crew members should be prepared with their own food and water (eating from the aid stations is usually prohibited), chairs, something to keep them occupied, and clothing appropriate for the expected (and unexpected) weather conditions. For hundred-milers, the crew should also be prepared to take turns sleeping through the night by having a somewhat comfortable resting place.

Crew Chief

I always like to appoint a crew chief that will be responsible for major decisions. This should be the person that is either the most experienced ultrarunner, most familiar with you as a runner, or the most levelheaded. A combination of all three is ideal. The crew chief will delegate responsibilities to other crew members, assess the state of the runner, and make final decisions in the likely event the runner is too tired or fatigued to think clearly. The crew chief should also be the person to make a final decision about the runner dropping from a race. If you do DNF (or finish the race), the crew chief is usually responsible for assuring your post-race celebratory beer isn't a *light* variety. That shit has no place in ultramarathons.

Crew Meeting

Before the race, the runner and crew should discuss pertinent issues. The runner should have a plan in place for aid station strategies, what clothing options he or she will have at each aid station, possible shoe changes, if he or she will need a light at a particular place, and anything else that is relevant. The runner should discuss the expected pace based on the race goals. The runner should also discuss contingency plans. For example, if the runner plans on a sub-twenty-four hour pace, what happens if the runner experiences trouble? Do he or she have a backup goal? Will the runner be satisfied with a finish even if he or she dead last and finishes a few minutes before the cutoff?

It's also important to discuss situations that will result in the runner dropping from the race. Most runners dramatically underestimate the depth of the lows they will experience. *There will be a point where you will want to quit.* Discuss how the crew should handle this.

My preference is to keep going unless I have a serious injury that threatens life or limb. I'm usually happy with finishing ultras no matter how slow. I have a pretty hearty ego and don't mind finishing dead last. I've finished races after sustaining minor injuries that required twenty to thirty miles of walking. I also know most lows are temporary and instruct my crew to ignore my plea to drop if it only occurs at one or two aid stations. If I'm in a sustained low for more than a marathon, I'll usually drop.

When the crew meets the runner, members should have a checklist of things to do. I like my crews to do the following:

- **Make sure they (or a volunteer) refill my water bottles.**
- **Remind me to get rid of any trash I may be carrying (remember, littering is a big no-no).**
- **Remind me to eat; tell me what foods the aid station has available.** This is important because aid stations don't always have all food choices readily available. Almost all use tables, but some stuff will spoil if exposed to warm temperatures for too long.
- **Ask me about chafing and remind me to lube up.** Nothing ruins a race faster than a chafed Johnson.
- **Ask me how my feet are doing; have new shoes and socks ready should I need to change.** I'll also have them help with untying if it's later in the race and I can't bend over.
- **Have a change of clothes ready and alert me of any weather changes in the immediate future.** If I'm wearing a spaghetti-strap tank top and there's an approaching snowstorm, they have to remind me to change.

- **Give me my flashlight and backup headlamp if it is close to dark, or take the lights if it's past sunrise.** If it's in the middle of the night, I may have them change batteries.
- **Have a chair ready if I need to sit down.** This can be dangerous; sitting tends to add significant time to aid station stops. However, some maintenance requires sitting (like feet).
- **Cheer me up by making bad jokes.** Luckily my friends have a dark sense of humor that rivals my own. Off-color jokes play well at 4 a.m.
- **Provide boobs.** Shelly has been known to flash me during particularly low points. While it's not something all crews need to do, it's worth considering. Boobs can be a powerful motivator. The more gender-conscious readers may be asking "What about Shelly?" She appreciates a good flash, too.

RUNNING BECOMES OUR LIVES

After the Burning River hundred-mile finish, our lives started to get crazy. Up to that point, Shelly and I were just high school teachers that dabbled in running. School had started. My crappy book had sold fairly well, and I was in the process of making a better version. I was determined to continue running ultras and solving this giant puzzle with the goal of eventually tackling a mountain hundred-miler. It seemed innocent enough. Little did I know our lives would be completely flipped upside down within the next nine months.

I had been writing minimalist shoe reviews on my Barefoot Running University website for a few years (good way to get free shoes), and had contacted Merrell, an outdoor company that was preparing to release a line of minimalist shoes. I didn't know it at the time, but my friend Angie Hotz (Barefoot Angie Bee) had dropped my name as a potential consultant to help the company develop educational material to distribute with their shoes. Instead of just sending me a pair of shoes, Meg Hammond from their marketing department wanted to meet in person. I had a barefoot clinic that week at a local Crossfit gym, so I invited her.

The clinic night came around and I went through my normal preparatory routine. I had set up my now sizable collection of traditional and minimalist shoes, had diagrams and graphs drawn on the dry erase board, and had free copies of the new edition of my book set out.

Meg was the first to show up. We chatted for a bit. I gave her a rundown of my background; she explained Merrell's foray into minimalism. During a lull in the conversation, I glanced at the clock. The clinic was supposed to have started fifteen minutes earlier.

Nobody showed up.

Every other clinic had at least ten to fifteen participants. Needless to say it was embarrassing. Still, Meg seemed impressed with the work I had been doing. I was impressed with the research they had done before producing the shoe. It was apparent they were committed to this new idea of minimalism. She was interested in using me as a consultant and this could be an opportunity to reach a bigger audience. She then gave me a pair of their flagship "barefoot" shoe, the Trail Glove. I tried them on. I walked around a bit. She asked what I thought. I replied, "They're pretty good."

I lied.

The shoes felt terrible. The fit felt strange. They hugged my feet in weird places. The sole wasn't entirely flat, so part of the shoe was touching the arch of my foot. I suddenly had a dilemma: I really didn't like this stupid shoe, but this could be an opportunity to reach people I could never reach before and play a role in changing the running industry. I resisted the urge to tell her "Thanks but no thanks." Instead, I asked to meet with the rest of the marketing team.

I left the meeting with conflicting emotions. I decided to give it a few days to fully process all the details. The next day, I decided to try the crappy-ass shoes on an actual trail run. I drove to the trailhead, laced up the shoes, and headed out. I usually walk as a warm-up, and the shoes felt exactly as they did the night before—*bad*.

Then I started to run.

I was immediately blown away. The shoe suddenly came alive. That weird fit allowed my foot to move perfectly within the shoe while still remaining in place. That "arch support" compressed and allowed the arch of my foot to function as if I were barefoot. Best of all, the sole provided the perfect combination of ground feel (how well I could feel the stuff under foot) and protection. At that point, I had tried maybe thirty to forty minimalist shoes, and this one was the best *by a long shot*.

I went home and sent Meg a long, rambling email. That started my formal relationship with the company. Over the next few months, my tasks grew from writing blog posts for the Merrell blog to writing educational content for their website, to eventually shooting instructional videos with Jon Sanregret and Sloan Dorr.

The day we were shooting the *barefoot* videos immediately after an unusually early snowstorm, I got a voicemail from Shelly. She was *really* excited, but didn't give details in the message. The Western States Endurance Run lottery was being held that day, and I knew she was watching online. I had qualified by finishing Burning River and entered the lottery on a drunken whim. The race is sometimes called the "Superbowl" of ultras, but I didn't have much interest in the race because I assumed it was out of my league. There were rumors the race committee was making the selection process more difficult after wildfires canceled the event the year before, which sparked my interest in entering the lottery.

I called her back as soon as we took a break from shooting. I was picked! The euphoria quickly morphed into anxiety as I realized I would need to do some serious training. My previous two ultras were run on relatively flat courses with rolling hills, fairly smooth trails, and close to sea level. Western starts in Squaw Valley, California, near Lake Tahoe, then follows the Western States trail through the Sierra Nevada Mountains down to the town of Auburn, California.

I spent the next few days mapping out exactly what I would have to do to successfully train for the race. I used everything I had learned before. I knew the race couldn't be run barefoot as Leif Rustvold had previously suffered through the race in Vibram Five Fingers. Luckily the Merrell Trail Gloves were proving to get even better once they broke in. I would be ready for this beast! *Or so I thought.*

The next five months turned out to be the busiest of my life. Shelly and I were teaching full-time. I was our union's vice president. We now had three children. I was maintaining a five-blog-posts-per-week writing pace. I was writing content for Merrell. My book was self-published, which included having to pick up physical copies at the local printer, storing them in my basement, then sending them out when ordered. I managed to squeeze in the occasional long run, but had ceased weight training and speedwork.

The real bombshell occurred when I was meeting with Merrell and happened to mention we were considering doing some RV travel that summer after Western States. A few days later, Merrell asked if we would be interested in doing some clinics at various retailers over the summer since we were traveling anyway. Shelly and I loved the idea! It would help fund the trip and give me a chance to do clinics outside the greater West Michigan area.

At this point, Shelly and I were becoming disillusioned with the education field. No Child Left Behind was quickly eroding our autonomy to the point where it felt like we were glorified tutors. The state budget cuts were increasing our class sizes while gouging our pay and benefits. We started exploring the logistics of moving to another state or even another profession. My book was doing far better than expected, so we had a regular income. We mentioned this to Merrell. A few days later, they gave us a proposal: we would travel the country full-time while holding running clinics at Merrell retailers.

The idea was scary as hell. We were considering leaving our tenured teaching positions that featured good benefits and a nice pension plan and the accompanying suburban lifestyle to become nomadic RV-dwelling hobos. With three kids. As scary as it was, we knew it would be a once-in-a-lifetime opportunity.

We decided to do it.

The logistics of planning added to the already-packed schedule. We used the book money to pay off debt and buy our "tow vehicle," a giant Chevy Suburban with an 8.1 liter V8. We needed something that, despite the seven miles per gallon gas mileage, would pull the trailer up mountain passes. We researched and found a suitable RV, a thirty-four-foot travel trailer with four bunks in the back. Throughout this entire process, we had one nagging issue: we wouldn't have access to a regular babysitter. We solved this problem by convincing our niece Stephanie to travel with us. She could watch the kids while we did clinics, races, or went on training runs. Everything was coming together nicely.

Except training for Western States.

I ran a handful of races, including the frigid Huff 50k in Indiana, the Mind the Ducks twelve hour (where I was hampered with severe diarrhea that turned out to be a pain in the ass), and the Pineland Farms fifty-miler in Maine. None of those races went well. The stress of being inadequately prepared for the biggest race of my life was conveniently overshadowed by the stress of completely uprooting our lives.

Eventually the school year ended, which was sad . . . it was hard leaving our students. We pushed back our "hit the road" date until after Western States in order to give us a buffer to give away our remaining possessions. In that interim, we flew to an event in Boulder, Colorado. Jesse Scott was spending the summer in Boulder, so I had an opportunity to explore the local trails. This gave me a little bit of experience running at altitude, which would be required for the early stages of Western States. Jesse also gave me some great downhill running tips. Western is a net-downhill race, meaning you run downhill significantly more than you run uphill. Unfortunately, uphills were my relative strength. His tips were welcomed.

The race finally rolled around. My crew and pacers for the race consisted of Shelly, Jeremiah Cataldo, Mark Robillard, Michael Helton, and Brandon Mulnix, who had crewed and paced for our friend Roger Bonga at the race the year before. We arrived a few days early to soak up the atmosphere. Western is like no other race due to the historical significance of the event. It's like an ultrarunning carnival. We spent our time attending the clinics and meetings, doing light running on the local trails, and generally screwing around.

I didn't fully disclose my pessimism with my crew. My training had been abysmal. I was twenty pounds heavier than my Burning River weight the previous year. There was an incredibly strong likelihood I was going to DNF this race. My goal was to simply see as much of the historic course as I could.

Before the race, Brandon decided to crew and pace for a runner that didn't have a crew or pacer. It worked out well, as I had more than enough support with Shelly, Jeremiah, Michael, and Mark. During our prerace meetings, it was decided that Jeremiah would do the brunt of the pacing given he was the fastest and most sadistic (good qualities in a pacer). Shelly would close it out based on her ability to get me to run the previous year at Burning River. I didn't tell them I had serious doubts I'd be able to make it far enough to even need a pacer.

Race morning came quickly. When preparing my gear, I purposely "forgot" my watch and grabbed my small point-and-shoot camera. I didn't want to know how slow I was going and I wanted pictures to remember the event.

The start line was abuzz with nervous energy. There were people everywhere. There were news and film crews. Our room was only about a hundred yards from the start line, which was convenient. About fifteen minutes before the start, I wandered to the starting corral. Amid the roar of cowbells and screams, we counted down to the start. A cannon signified the beginning of the race.

Western begins with several miles of climbing up to Emigrant Pass. I was busy snapping pictures and chatting with James Barstad, a friend I had met previously at Burning River.

As we neared the top of Emigrant Pass, we hit the first significant snow. Even though it was June, it had been an unusually heavy snow year. The course's alternative "snow route" even had to be modified. This worked to my advantage given I ran *a lot* of snowy trails in Michigan.

I spent the entire first forty or so miles blissfully snapping away pictures and soaking in the amazing scenery. I had no idea how fast I was going, only that I was somewhere ahead of the thirty-hour cutoff. I was having a blast, though. I was in a joking mood the entire time. Western is known for the fabulous aid stations, all of which are staffed by experienced ultrarunners, amazing food, and many medical professionals. At one point, a volunteer doctor asked me if I needed anything. I scratched my junk and asked "Ya got anything for crabs?"

The crew had split up due to the transit time between the Michigan Bluff and Foresthill aid stations, so I met Mark and Michael first. As I came into the aid station, I saw Brandon first. That surprised me as Brandon had spent days bragging about his runner being faster than me. Both Mark and Michael repeatedly told me I was doing great. I assumed they meant I was under the cutoff. I spent a little too much time at the aid station mostly because, due to the snow, this was the first time my crew could reach me. I eventually got up and continued toward the next aid station.

I continued to snap pictures and enjoy the run. When I got to the Foresthill aid station, Jeremiah and Shelly came out to meet me before I entered the actual aid station (crew was not allowed inside). They were *way* more excited than they usually were, which I understood when they told me I wasn't just under the thirty-hour cutoff pace. I was forty-five minutes over the twenty-four hour pace! By willingly ignoring any measure of my performance, I was doing better than I ever had before.

Western States is one of the few ultras that gives a different award for finishing under a particular time, and the silver cougar buckle is one of ultrarunning's most coveted prizes. I had dreamed about the possibilities of earning one way back in the days following the lottery, but my total lack of preparation quickly dashed all hope. Until that very moment. I had about thirty-eight miles to make up forty-five minutes. I knew it would be nearly impossible because I'm not a very good runner, but I also knew I had phenomenal pacers in Jeremiah and Shelly, and Michael and Mark were experienced crew members. If I were going to do it, this was the crew that could get me there.

Jeremiah did an excellent job of pushing me when needed, instructing me when to eat and drink, and generally doing everything a great pacer is supposed to do. By this point in my ultra career, I had figured out that I could minimize the low points by consuming enough calories. Indeed, Jeremiah kept me from bonking until about mile ninety. I told the crew to continue keeping in the dark regarding time as it turned out to be a great motivator. As such, I didn't know if I had made up time or not. Based on Jeremiah and the rest of the crew's demeanor, I knew I was close.

Too close.

Somewhere in the night, we met the crew. My Fenix handheld flashlight batteries were dying, and it took special lithium batteries. Regular alkaline batteries wear out quickly, usually within about two hours. Someone was supposed to have the batteries ready. When we pulled into the aid station, either Mark or Michael handed me the alkalines. I handed them back and said I needed the lithiums. I went back to eating and restocking my water bottle pockets with gels. I grabbed my flashlight and it was too light. There were no batteries in it. Mark and Michael were standing next to each other chatting. I *may* have frantically screamed something about needing "the damn lithiums!"

I'm still not quite sure how the incident went down as my sleep-derived memories are sketchy. Regardless, I'm pretty sure I was a complete jackass. I felt terrible. They were, after all, volunteering their time to help me. It was the last time I ever yelled at my crew or volunteers.

When I could, I pounded a Red Bull and ate as much as I could stomach. Sure enough, I pulled out of the low. As we headed into the Highway 49 aid station at about mile ninety-three, I asked Jeremiah if he thought I should pick Shelly up to pace as planned. At that point, Shelly had never run trails in the dark. When I made the plan I hadn't anticipated running this section at night. He was noncommittal but indicated he *could* do it.

When we arrived at the aid station, the discussion was quick. I believe the dialogue went something like this:

Me: "You've never run trails at night, are you sure you want to do it? Jeremiah said he can pace me the rest of the way."

Shelly (while grabbing her water bottle and exiting the aid station): "Get your ass moving!"

It was a quick discussion.

Shelly didn't let up that entire section. Based on her frantic pushing, I assumed I was still very close. We filled each other in on the previous day. I told her about the joy of running in the snow-covered high country and the switchbacks going down then back up the canyons. She told me about the dumbass shenanigans the crew was doing while waiting. It was basically a date night, only I smelled really bad.

Eventually we reached the illuminated "No Hands Bridge" crossing the American River. This was the second-to-the-last aid station. For the first time, I knew I was going to finish *no matter what*. That's a great feeling in a hundred-miler. I still didn't know how I was doing on time, but Shelly seemed more relaxed at this aid station. I was a little frantic trying to eat some orange slices when a volunteer chuckled and said "Calm down son, choking on the orange is the only thing that will keep you from getting that silver buckle."

That's when I knew we had done it. We still had three point four miles to go and I didn't want to take chances. We quickly exited the aid station and crossed the bridge. It really was a beautiful moment and I was glad I was able to share it with Shelly.

I continued to run as hard as I could, though it was mostly uphill. We arrived at the final aid station, Robie Point, with somewhere around forty minutes to go. The final mile or so is run through a residential section of Auburn. My entire crew could run with me at this point, so they enjoyed taunting me as I tried to muster a running pace. As we neared the Placer High School track, the end of the race, I could see the floodlights and hear the PA announcer. We entered the gate to the track and started the halflap to the finish. Two people "sprinted" past me as I slowed my pace. I was going to make it under twenty-four hours and had plenty of time to spare. I was going to enjoy the last two hundred meters of the best race I had ever run.

I crossed the finish line around 23:40. I hugged my crew, allowed the medical crew to do their checks (a rarity in the ultra world), then limped to the car. We were heading to Denny's!

From what I remember, the service was terrible, I ate some sort of egg dish, and apparently fell asleep at the table.

For those that like a visual reference, here's a dorky video montage of the experience:
www.youtube.com/watch?v=-OkZDAI3YiQ.

Western States was a game changer for me. Previously, I had mostly relied on mixing and matching conventional wisdom from experienced ultrarunners. Based on that conventional wisdom, I should not have finished Western States let alone finished under twenty-four hours. I had clearly done something right, but what?

Was it the low-volume training? Maybe it was the lack of pressure of maintaining a pace. Or it could have been looking at the race as an opportunity to take pictures and explore. Was it my expert crew and pacers? There were just so many potential variables. I knew I had to run at least one more hundred-miler to see if I could replicate the results.

We returned to Michigan and prepared to leave on our RV adventure. I checked our schedule and cross-referenced it with possible races. Grindstone, a hundred-miler in Virginia, fit perfectly. The race would be significantly more difficult than Western States, but that shiny silver buckle gave me a huge confidence boost. I signed up the night before we left Michigan.

SECTION 7:
TRAINING FOR ULTRAMARATHONS

LEARNING WHEN THINGS ARE ABOUT TO GO BAD

This material is mostly redundant, but important enough to restate. This is the crux of ultrarunning: *learning to solve problems that arise*. When training in various bodily states, you get to experiment with quite a few different variables. Another significant advantage is learning to recognize the early signs of significant issues that plague ultrarunners. Here are some examples:

- **Glycogen or carbohydrate depletion:** As discussed earlier, your body has a finite number of carbs to fuel your muscles. When the supply runs low, your body has to convert fat as a fuel source, which is a significantly slower process of delivering fuel to working muscles. This usually results in a crash or hitting "the wall," which is one of the most common causes of runners dropping out of a race. Learning how this feels is among the most valuable skills you can learn. If you begin experiencing the early signs, consuming something sugary can prevent the crash.

- **Dehydration:** For me, recognizing the bodily sensations of early dehydration is difficult. Instead, I rely on other signs. I use urine frequency and color. If I'm peeing at least once every two hours and the urine color is clear or light yellow (like lemonade), I know I'm good. If I'm peeing less frequently or my urine is darker color (like apple juice), I know I'm nearing dehydration and will start drinking more. It's not an exact science, but still pretty effective. What about at night? I just shine a headlamp through the stream to determine color. Practice it a few times. What about women? This answer comes from Shelly: she recommends learning to pee standing up (as opposed to squatting) and, like my suggestion, use a headlamp through the stream to determine color. Again, practice the technique. The technique also works well at truck stop bathrooms.

- **Sleep deprivation:** Sleep deprivation is a major issue for me as evident by the previous sections, but usually only in longer races. If I'm excessively sleep deprived, my mood turns negative. I'm far more likely to stop a race due to sleep deprivation than anything else. The problem is sleep deprivation symptoms can be similar to glycogen depletion. Sleep deprivation is somewhat tricky because the best fix is actually sleeping. Loading up on stimulants may be a temporary fix (like pounding a Red Bull or taking a few hits off the crack pipe). If that solution doesn't work, it is possible to counteract some of the effects with a fifteen-minute power nap.

- **Hyponatremia:** This is a life-threatening condition that is caused by too little sodium in your body. It usually results from consuming too much water and not enough sodium. Some symptoms are weight gain and swelling. The prevention is simple: take supplemental electrolytes during runs, especially if it is hot. I prefer Succeed S-Caps and will take one about every hour or two. Consuming sports drinks instead of straight water can also be useful.

TRAINING PARTNERS

Before we get to the nuts and bolts of experimentation ideas, let's chat about training partners. Some people are attracted to ultras for the solitude when training. Or, as was my case, you're looking for a little peace and quiet from your screaming newborn. If this is you, there's no need for a training partner or partners . . . enjoy the silence.

For those of you that prefer a more social setting, finding good training partners can be invaluable. I have the benefit of having an ultrarunning spouse. In fact, many of the "dates" Shelly and I go on involve running up and down mountains. We also have a great network of friends collectively known as the "Hobby Joggas." We routinely go on group runs then hit up a local bar afterward.

Here are some tips to find training partners:

Tip #1: Find other ultrarunners. Social networking is great for this. Facebook is teeming with runners; many probably live near you. Connecting with them is easy, and most arc always looking for new training partners. It's also a great way to get advice from those that have more experience.

Tip #2: Convince your friends to join you on this adventure. If your friends are adventurous, they'll probably join with little hesitation. If they are not adventurous, just lie by omission. If you're training for a 50k, tell them you're training for a 5k and just start going through the training plan. At some point they will catch on. At that point, just say "Oh, did I say *5k*, I meant *50k*! I've always had trouble with zeros."

Tip #3: Get a dog that likes to run. They make great training partners. I'd suggest some sort of sled dog breed. I used to own a Pomeranian, which is apparently a descendant of sled dogs. Once trained, he could easily run twenty-plus miles as long as the temperatures were cool. Other active breeds will work, too. Avoid dogs like bulldogs as they aren't well-suited for running. Avoid little dogs like miniature pinschers, wiener dogs, or Chihuahuas, too. That just looks silly.

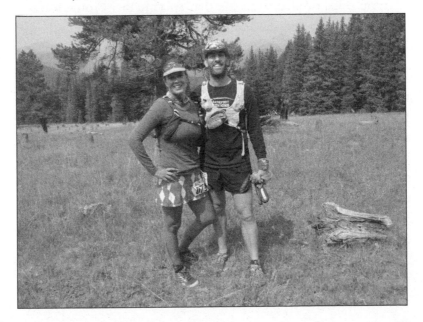

COURSE-SPECIFICITY TRAINING

If you have the opportunity to practice on the ultra course, take it! Being familiar with the course is a huge advantage. Not only do you learn the useful information like aid station locations and potential trouble spots but you also will be developing the running skills needed to tackle that specific race. You'll learn to run through the specific rocks, roots, mud holes, and hills that litter the course.

In the event you cannot run the same course, try to find a place to train that is as similar to the course as possible. Match up things like altitude, elevation change, surface (hard-packed dirt, gravel, sand, rock, etc.).

Early in my ultra career, I rarely had the opportunity to train on the course I was planning on running. I did go to great lengths to find comparable trails, though. This usually involved scouring YouTube and Google Images for any visuals I could find. It also involved reading as many race reports as I could find.

Some variables are nearly impossible to experience, like altitude. When I trained for Western States (with a maximum altitude of 11,000 feet), I needed a way to simulate the lack of oxygen I'd experience. I lived in Michigan, which has an altitude of about 500 feet above sea level. The solution? I did several runs while breathing through a drinking straw from McDonald's. While I doubt it did anything physiologically, it did teach me a valuable lesson: there was a definite connection between available oxygen and pace. I quickly learned to be especially conservative and take frequent walk breaks. I also learned our local police department is suspicious of dudes running barefoot at night while breathing through a straw. What's weird about that?

RACING AS TRAINING

Running shorter races can be an excellent method of training for ultras. The races act as a quality training run and allow you to go through your prerace routine. If the race is shorter, like a 5k, it will serve as good speedwork. If it is longer, like a half marathon, it will serve as a good long run.

Another great technique is to do a long run by running a race course prior to the race, then running the race afterward. I learned this technique from my friend Phil Stapert. He uses this idea to train for hundred-milers.

This method can be especially useful if the race is run on the same course as your ultra. Check with the race director or the race website. They will usually be familiar with other races run on the same trails or roads.

SLEEP-DEPRIVATION TRAINING

Mark "Doc" Ott wrote a blog post about his strategy for ultra training: *www.docott.com/run/?m=201209.*

He came up with a method that allows him to hit high mileage and still spend time with his family.

His methodology brought back not-so-fond memories of my early days as an ultrarunner. I was more or less in the same boat—I had a finite amount of time to train but needed to build an endurance base to handle the rigors of ultramarathons. My solution was similar to his: wake up ridiculously early in the morning (2 to 3 a.m.), run, get ready for work, drop kids off at day care, work, pick kids up, engage in family time, put kids to bed, spend time with Shelly, go running again, sleep.

I did this for about a year. It served the purpose; I built a pretty good endurance base that has persisted for years. I also got a pretty decent string of sleep-deprivation training runs since we had two babies that woke up throughout the night.

My experiences in hundred-milers with this sleep-deprivation training was mixed. I didn't get especially tired until after 4 a.m. I didn't get deliriously tired until sunrise, and the feeling persisted for about two hours. This wasn't a major issue until the 2011 Grindstone 100 when a 6 p.m. start coupled with a variety of other issues that led to a DNF.

I was determined to find a better method for overcoming sleep deprivation. The applicable science is pretty straightforward. We normally have a twenty-four-hour sleep-wake cycle, which is one of many circadian cycles that regulate bodily processes. If we have a fairly predictable wake-up time, our body quickly adapts to specific periods of sleep and wakefulness. We have the ability to manipulate the sleep-wake cycle. If we stayed awake for twenty-four hours at a time, we'd eventually adapt to that sleep-wake cycle. Unfortunately we're continually confounded by the sun. We have light-sensitive photoreceptor cells in our eyes that reset our internal clocks each day. Besides, those pesky "jobs" usually prevent unusual sleep-wake cycles.

The other biological issue is our biological need for sleep. We can't live without sleep. Literally. If we lose the ability to sleep, we die. A chemical called adenosine builds up in our bloodstream when we're awake. The longer we're awake, the more adenosine builds up. This chemical makes us feel sleepy, impairs cognitive function, and negatively affects coordination and balance, along with a host of other undesirable effects that sabotage running.

Caffeine, the world's most popular psychoactive drug, works by temporarily blocking adenosine. One option in ultras is to drink a shit ton of caffeinated beverages. Indeed, Red Bull and Monster are staples of my hundred-miler drop bags. Unfortunately the effects are short-lived and result in a crashing effect after the adenosine-blocking wears off. You feel even more tired than you would if you hadn't consumed caffeine.

The other option is sleep, which dissipates adenosine. Interestingly, it doesn't take much sleep for this effect to occur. A fifteen-minute power nap should result in a significant reduction of adenosine. That's the biological basis for the power nap. It's long enough to affect adenosine but short enough to prevent us from slipping into the deeper stages of sleep that make us feel groggy upon waking. The problem: lying down and remaining immobile for fifteen minutes at mile seventy almost always results in severe stiffness (not the morning-wood type) and possibly exercise-induced cramping.

My Tested Solutions

I knew the two-a-day runs were not quite as effective as they needed to be based on Grindstone. I had a great opportunity to test a few different strategies at the seventy-two-hour Across the Years race last December. I tried the fifteen-minute power nap, a ninety-minute sleep period (to theoretically go through all five stages of sleep), and several variations of multiples of ninety-minute sleep periods (three hours, four and a half hours, six hours).

I found four and a half worked well. Three hours was too short, as was ninety minutes. Unfortunately that didn't help much for hundos. There's no way I could give up four and a half hours by sleeping. I'm not fast enough to create a large buffer for cutoff times. That essentially put me back to square one.

The Accidental Solution

Around late winter, Shelly and I decided to alter our travel methods. When we first hit the road and we had a long distance between clinics, we would break up the drive into six- to seven-hour blocks. A drive halfway across the country might take us four days. Those travel days sucked because our kids were stir-crazy when we stopped. It took forever to calm them down. We decided to experiment with driving these routes in one block—through the night.

At first it was tough. I would stop several times for the aforementioned power nap. After three or four such trips, I noticed my night endurance increasing. I felt less drowsy. I had to stop less. I consumed less caffeine.

I didn't really consider the effects on hundos until Bighorn. The race was an 11 a.m. start, which guaranteed I'd be running through the night and well into the following day. Indeed, the race took me over thirty-two hours. Much to my surprise, I made it through the night with minimal sleep-deprivation symptoms. I immediately made the driving connection.

The theory was sort of tested again at the Grand Mesa 100. Shelly and I ended up DNFing, but not before we got a healthy dose of night running. Again, I had very few sleep-deprivation symptoms. The system seemed to work. Practicing staying awake for large blocks of time actually helps you stay awake for large blocks of time.

Conclusion

So . . . what would I recommend for sleep-deprivation training?

Stay up all night occasionally. I do it about once monthly. Since it is tough physiologically, I don't recommend doing it more often.

I still question exactly why it was so effective. Did it cause my body to physiologically adapt to an occasional lack of sleep? Or am I simply learning to deal with the symptoms of sleep deprivation, thus reducing their severity? Or was it just a placebo effect and I just believe I can handle it better? Regardless, it is effective.

FASTING WHILE TRAINING

Many of my ultra friends have started experimenting with low heart rate training. The technique is based on the idea that we can train our body to run faster while remaining in an aerobic zone (burning fat versus carbs as a primary fuel). Many people have had success with the method. I've played around with the idea but found the long, slow running to be too boring. *It took the fun out of running.*

For years, I've used a *different* technique that accomplishes a similar task. I purposely fast about twelve to twenty-four hours before some of my long runs, then do not eat during the run. This forces glycogen depletion very early in the run. As a result, my body burns its available stockpile of carbs. At first, the crash is severe. It's what marathoners like to call "the wall." My average pace decreases dramatically and I feel terrible. After a few such runs, the crash becomes a lot less severe and I'm able to maintain a much faster post-crash pace. Furthermore, the subjective feeling evolves from "horrible" to "eh, this isn't too bad." In essence,

I'm training my body to deal with glycogen depletion and utilize fat as a primary fuel source.

With low heart rate training, the goal is to increase your aerobic pace to decrease finish times. This works well if you remain under that aerobic threshold, or the point where your body is using mostly fat as fuel, for the entire race. Personally I don't like to have that limitation. I like the freedom of adjusting my pace based on how I feel, the terrain, available food, competition . . . whatever.

Low heart rate training teaches your body to utilize fat as a fuel, which allows you to run faster while using more fat and less glycogen. Regularly training on an empty stomach does something similar. Check out these articles:

Piece of evidence #1: *www.marathonguide.com/training/articles/MandBFuelOnFat.cfm.*

Piece of evidence #2: *www.ncbi.nlm.nih.gov/pubmed/20452283.*

The Elite Question

People sometimes ask how elite ultrarunners race while consuming very little food. Here's an example. At the Bighorn Ultra in 2012, Damian Stoy (an accomplished ultrarunner, running form coach, and frutarian), the fifty-mile overall winner, ran the race on *three* gels. That's roughly 300 calories. He would have burned between 5,000–6,000 calories for the entire race. Assuming he started with about 2,000 calories worth of glycogen (stored in muscles and the liver), he would have had at least a 2,700 calorie deficit over the course of the race. Most of those 2,700 calories had to come from fat.

How is it he could have maintained a winning pace (9:22) over rugged terrain with lots of climbing while fighting a glycogen deficit? He had to rely on fat as fuel. But he clearly wasn't running below his aerobic threshold (he was breathing hard when he passed me). I would hypothesize that he does what most fast runners tend to do—*eat very little before and during training runs.*

What Would I Recommend?

Low heart rate training is an invaluable tool . . . for building a good endurance base. The low intensity dramatically decreases recovery time and limits the occurrence of injuries. I highly recommend new runners use this method to build an endurance base regardless of your goal distances.

Once you build that base, however, low heart rate training is of little value. The slow pace will limit your speed. Doing speedwork like fartlek runs, tempo runs, and interval training will help make you faster. If you're planning to run anything over a half marathon, adding foodless training will continue to develop your ability to use fat as fuel. This will limit the negative effects of the "wall" that cripples so many runners.

Let's look at a typical marathoner. Most marathon training plans top out at around twenty- to twenty-two-mile long runs. If a marathoner eats before a long run of that distance, it's unlikely they will experience glycogen depletion during training. When running the actual race, they cross that line of glycogen depletion during those last few miles. Since it's something their body rarely if ever experiences, it hits hard. Really, really hard.

You can eliminate this problem using a few methods:

- **Run the entire race below your aerobic threshold so you burn mostly fat.** This would be the strategy recommended by the low heart rate crowd. The problem? You're forced to stay below that threshold or you'll hit the wall.
- **Eat enough to cover the deficit.** In the case of a marathon, consuming 300 to 800 calories before or during the race will be enough to supply enough calories to cover that deficit. Personally I like this strategy, but it will fail if you can't eat enough to cover the distance.
- **Train to run despite the wall.** By training regularly on an empty stomach and purposely hitting the wall, you'll limit the negative effects of glycogen depletion.

The best-case scenario would be to utilize all three. Build an endurance base using low heart rate training. During the race, eat if you can. If you can't, foodless training will guarantee performance won't be impeded by a glycogen crash.

The Actual Training

I try to use this method at least twice per week. It's pretty easy—just run long enough to deplete your glycogen stores. The longer you fast before your run, the earlier you'll crash. If I eat immediately before a run, I'll usually hit the wall around mile eighteen to twenty. If I fast for twelve hours, it usually hits around thirteen to fifteen. If I fast for twenty-four hours, I may hit the wall within the first five to eight miles. Your results will vary. Once you hit the crash, continue running for a few miles without eating. I aim for about four to five miles.

The first few times are going to be awful. Your pace will decrease dramatically. You'll feel drained. Stuff will hurt. You'll probably feel depressed. Don't worry; all of these symptoms will ease after a few training sessions. Eventually the "crash" barely registers. Furthermore, each subsequent crash experienced in the same run is lessened. In an ultra, this is important because most people decide to drop from races while in the middle of an especially bad low point. Make the low points more tolerable and your finish rate increases.

This method also teaches you to predict when glycogen depletion is about to occur. You'll learn the subtle, often-missed early signs mentioned in the previous paragraph. In a race, these signs can be used as a cue to eat something, thus preventing the crash before it becomes worse.

I like to do these training sessions a few months before my goal race. Four or five sessions seems to produce good results. Eight to ten sessions seems to maximize the effect.

Conclusion

Training on an empty stomach can be an invaluable tool to your training if you plan to run longer races. It's not difficult (though mildly unpleasant in the beginning). The potential benefits can be huge as it frees you from the shackles of maintaining an aerobic-zone pace and regular food consumption. Personally this method has been instrumental in my own training for hundred-mile races.

GLUTTONY TRAINING

Before I get to the details, I should note this training really only applies to ultrarunners. Most people should be able to run anything up to about eighteen to twenty miles without any food. Even a marathon would require very little food, if any at all. Once you pass that marathon threshold, food becomes increasingly important as distance increases.

Many runners hit a point during a race where they simply cannot stomach any food. Either they don't have an appetite or the taste/smell of food makes them nauseous. As a result, they stop eating. This leads to a glycogen-depletion crash. That often leads to a DNF. The solution is simple: *train to eat.*

This is what I do. Approximately once every two or three weeks, I'll eat a fairly large meal about thirty minutes before a long run. My preferred meal is a quarter-pounder extra value meal. If you're fast food averse, any food will work . . . just make sure it's voluminous. On the same run, eat something about every thirty minutes. I'd shoot for 100 calories in the beginning, and slowly work up to 200–300 on subsequent runs. I like to experiment with the actual food to help figure out what foods I can tolerate. As the distance increases, your tastes will likely change.

This is invaluable information as it will help you pack drop bags for future ultras. Eventually you'll probably find a few foods that work in all situations. I always like to have these foods on-hand in races. My all-purpose foods are:

- Chia seeds
- Slimfast
- Turkey and cheese sandwiches
- Mashed potatoes

I can eat all four in any condition (i.e., they never make me nauseous). The key to this training is to go slow. If you feel like vomiting (which is normal in the beginning), slow down to a walk. Speed up when you feel better.

So what exactly are the benefits of this training?

- Appears to help teach your body to digest food better while running, which allows you to consume more calories per hour if and when it's needed
- Teaches you which foods you can tolerate while running
- Teaches you the skill of physically putting food in your mouth while moving
- Allows you to occasionally indulge in foods with little guilt (important for my foodie friends)
- Helps you develop a feel for how much you can eat and still perform well (too little = crash, too much = nausea)

I'd put this specific training method in the category of "unorthodox." However, it is effective. When I started running, I couldn't even eat a gel. Now I could consume a Thanksgiving dinner. This specific skill is easy to develop and has become a relative strength in races. I find it's usually better to eat too little instead of too much, but I know I can quickly and easily recover from a caloric deficit if needed. It's a handy tool to have in the toolbox.

USING HEART RATE AS A TRAINING TOOL

If you chose the Maffetone Method in the "Give Me a Training Plan!" section, you'll become intimately familiar with heart rate monitors. Even if you didn't, a heart rate monitor could be a valuable tool. Not only is it cool to see your heart rate in real time, it can be used as a great training tool to prepare your body for ultras.

The idea goes something like this: if you run slow enough, your body will burn primarily fat instead of carbohydrates. Since most of us have well over 100,000 "fat" calories stored in our bodies and only a few thousand "carb" calories, it makes sense to burn the fat. Besides that, the "bonk" or "wall" marathoners complain about is caused by your bodily supply of carbohydrates running low.

It's actually really easy to train your body to burn fat. Here are two ideas:

First, run your long runs slow. This is where a heart rate monitor comes into play. If you keep your heart rate low (here's Maffetone's formula: *www.philmaffetone.com/180formula.cfm*) on your long runs, you'll train your body to better utilize fat stores. There are other possible positive benefits, but this is a biggie.

Second, do at least a few of your runs after fasting. Don't eat for twelve to twenty-four hours prior to the run. You will reach the "wall" much faster as your body's supply of carbohydrates will be much lower. This isn't nearly as effective as the first technique, but it does familiarize you to the feelings associated with hitting that wall. If you experience the beginnings of those same feelings in a race, eating something sugary will usually reverse the effects. Knowing your body and the signals it's sending is important.

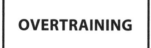

OVERTRAINING

Rest days are important. So much so, I'm placing this section ahead of the actual training ideas. When you decide to run an ultra, there's usually some degree of panic that sets in. It's not uncommon to have a *"Oh my God I'm not going to be ready for this!"* feeling. That sometimes drives us to train again and again without giving our bodies time to recover.

Most of the plans have built-in rest days. *Take them!* Your body needs that time to recover. If you don't rest, there's a chance you will develop overtraining symptoms, which include:

- A higher-than-normal heart rate, which can be measured when waking up in the morning (before those eight cups of coffee)
- Constant muscle soreness
- Insomnia
- Depression-like symptoms
- Loss of appetite
- Loss of motivation
- Irritability

The tricky part of diagnosing overtraining is that the symptoms are hard to distinguish from other negative life events, like your favorite reality TV show being canceled or your pet gerbil dying.

I've encountered overtraining occasionally. My challenge has been deciphering the symptoms of overtraining from my natural procrastination and laziness. For me the tell-tale sign is loss of appetite. It never happens. I once ate an entire large pepperoni pizza in the middle of a bout of the stomach flu. It wasn't pretty.

If you start experiencing overtraining symptoms, what's the best solution? *Take a one-week vacation.* No matter where you are in training, take a week off. Do nothing. The effects on training will be minimal and you'll come back stronger than ever.

TAPERING

Tapering is the process of resting prior to running a race. The idea is to train hard for a period of time, then give your body a chance to fully heal before you hit the start line. There are several schools of thought regarding tapering.

Some advocate a long, drawn-out taper where you slowly ramp down mileage and intensity. A common strategy is to begin the taper about a month before the race by reducing your training volume by about 50 percent each week, then eliminating running completely in the week immediately before the race. I used this strategy for my first three years of ultrarunning. Since my body wasn't quite adapted to the rigors of ultrarunning, it worked fairly well. I was healthy, but felt a little rusty for the first half of the race.

Eventually I moved toward the second school of thought—utilizing a very limited taper. I would maintain a normal training routine until about three days before a race, then do short "shake-out" runs each day. This strategy worked well because I didn't feel rusty the morning of the race.

Most beginners could probably utilize a middle ground strategy. Unless you're injured, there's not much of a need to taper for four weeks. Two weeks should be adequate for almost everyone. As you gain more experience, you can shorten the length of the taper.

CONQUERING THE HUNDRED-MILERS! OR NOT.

My relative success at Western States should have been a major boost to my ultrarunner ego. However, the combination of false confidence ("Damn, I'm good!) and misattribution ("I've been working hard all these years? Clearly less is more.") were terrible, which became painfully evident later that fall. I had signed up for the Grindstone hundred-miler in the Blue Mountains of Virginia, which was widely regarded as one of the most difficult hundred-milers east of the Mississippi.

Immediately after Western States, we returned to Michigan to finalize our preparation to hit the road. We gave away the last of our possessions, dropped off our mementos in a storage unit, and packed the few things we thought we would need. The day we actually left was surreal. We were literally driving away from our old life, yet it was decidedly unceremonious. We gave a few hugs, piled into the Suburban, and drove away.

We didn't have any clinics for awhile, so we traveled to our friend Scott Lucias's house in Ohio, then headed to the Laurel Highlands area of Pennsylvania. We were in explorer mode and wanted to discover new, interesting areas of our country. The RV lifestyle was pretty bizarre. The normal pressures of everyday life disappeared. Our days consisted of sleeping in when the kids allowed, leisurely enjoying breakfast, going for runs, teaching the kids (we were homeschooling at that point), or writing. We really were living the dream.

There are some obvious negatives of the RV lifestyle. In the spirit of full disclosure, the experience wasn't entirely muffins wrapped in rainbows. We had three adults and three children living in a three-hundred-square-foot area, so personal space was an issue. Everything was smaller, from the closet-like bathroom and tub/shower to the the small oven and refrigerator. Maintaining, and emptying, the gray water tank (bath and sink water) and black water tank (poopy water) took some acclimation. Let's just say there was an unfortunate "connector" issue the first time I emptied the black water tank at a Flying J somewhere in southeast Ohio.

There's also the sex issue, which was our most common question. Anyone that's ever spent a few minutes in an RV knows they shake. No matter how well they're stabilized, the tiniest movements are transmitted throughout. At first, we waited until we had alone time. That proved to be difficult because Stephanie could only take the kids to the park so many times. Then we resorted to waiting until everyone was asleep . . . or so we thought. At first we answered our kids' "why was the trailer shaking?" by blaming it on the wind. One day our oldest walked in on us and we had to explain what we were doing. We're pretty honest with our kids across the board, so it wasn't a major issue. Eventually they learned not to walk in on us when the accordion-like doors to our "bedroom" were shut. Minimally, we've assured they will have plenty of issues to discuss in therapy once they reach adulthood.

After we spent some time exploring the trails in Pennsylvania, we stopped in Ohio to reciprocate pacing and crewing duties for Jeremiah Cataldo as he ran the now-familiar Burning River 100. I was crewing and pacing with Dave Eaton, another gifted ultra-runner that had spent time in Kenya. The experience gave me the opportunity to pick his brain about training methods. I already knew Jeremiah's training included a great deal of fast running, and Dave's methodology was similar. That *should* have been a warning that my "lazy ass" training method wasn't what led to the decent Western States finish . . . but I'm stubborn.

After Burning River, we continued to travel, explore mountain trails, and even ran a marathon in Colorado and another in West Virginia. We also experienced one of the high points of our travels—the second annual (and now discontin-ued) New York City Barefoot Run. Friends John and Maggie Durant had organized the event to be the biggest barefoot and minimalist festival in the world. It drew a who's who of the mini-malist community including Dr. Dan Lieberman, Dr. Mark Cucuzzella, Esther Gokale, Ken Bob Saxton, Ted MacDonald, Chris McDougall, Dr. Daniel Howell, Erwan LeCorre, and Lee Saxby. It was an honor to be included in this group. Merrell sponsored the event and also planned a round table discussion that included the rest of the well-known and influential members of the community, which included many of my friends.

After the round table, we went to dinner and then attended a party. It was awesome to chat with hundreds of people that had a similar interest. They also had free beer. A few of us (Shelly, Jesse Scott, Christian Peterson, Kate Kift, Trisha Reeves, Pablo

Päster, and Krista Cavendar) ended up closing the bar (on the water in lower Manhattan) and wandered to our hotel four miles north. All of us were ridiculously drunk. I have no idea how we managed to navigate, though we took the subway at some point. Once we got back to our hotel, we hit the bar until somewhere around 3 a.m. Eventually we went to bed.

Jesse, Shelly, Pablo, and I overslept and missed the race which started the next morning. We eventually made it to the ferry to Governor's Island to join the festivities as they wound down. It was somewhat embarrassing to show up four hours late and still somewhat intoxicated. It was yet another indicator that we didn't take running nearly as seriously as some of our peers.

By the time the Grindstone 100 rolled around, I *thought* I was prepared. Jesse Scott and Shelly would serve as my crew and pacers, so I knew I was in good hands. The race started in the afternoon, which was a significant deviation from every other race I had ever ran. The race was also more rugged than any previous race. The rockiness of the trails rivaled the gnarliest trails we had encountered anywhere up to that point.

I woke up around 6 a.m. the day of the race. I'm a morning person, so it is difficult to sleep later. The race didn't start for another twelve hours, so I had a ton of time to kill. Jesse, Shelly, and I chatted about the race plans and strategy, ran some errands, then meandered to the camp that served as the start/finish line (the race is an out-and-back course). I tried taking a nap under some trees, but couldn't sleep. The nervous energy I had all day was starting to take a toll, but I tried to ignore it. About an hour before the race I started my normal prerace routine, which made me feel better. By the time the race started, I was feeling refreshed and ready.

The early stages of the race went well. I felt good, was eating and drinking, and found a comfortable gait. Around dark, I came upon a runner that was limping badly. I stopped to ask him if he was okay. Apparently he had fallen on a part of the trail that ran along a creek. He believed he had broken his femur, which sort of freaked me out. I offered to help carry him the mile or so to the next aid station, but he refused. I took his name and bib number and ran ahead to alert the aid station workers. The first two seemed rather dismissive, so I continued telling people until I found someone that would head back out to find him.

Once that excitement passed, I continued on to the first major climb. Going uphill has always been a strength, so I started a fast hike. The climb was several miles long and I felt awesome passing quite a few runners. Several complimented me on my uphill prowess, which inflated my ego even more. I got to the top, punched my race bib (the indicator that we made it to the turnaround point), then headed back down. The rough single track made it difficult to pass other runners, but I passed a few. There was a tiny voice in my head that warned me to slow down, but my post-Western States confidence silenced it. I was having some trouble eating my gels and running over the rough terrain in the dark, so I decided to wait until the trail smoothed out. Unfortunately I was having too much fun floating over the rocky trails in the dark to remember to keep eating.

The second climb started like the first—I was kicking ass. I was so busy dominating this supposedly "difficult" course I continued to neglect eating. The first big low hit on the descent from the second climb. As soon as I felt it start, I panicked. I realized I had completely neglected eating. I had enough experience to know what was coming. I frantically choked down all six Gu packets I was carrying. *That reminds me of a good ultrarunner tip: never eat six gels at one time!*

After I finished vomiting, I continued to panic. I had no food until the next aid station and I was on the cusp of a major low. I had no choice but to continue on. The low hit hard and I was forced to walk. I was still in a deep low when I hit the aid station. I ate a piece of candy and a small chunk of banana, grabbed another half dozen gels, and headed back out. I'd be meeting Shelly and Jesse at the next aid station, so I perked up a bit. That perkiness lasted about ninety seconds.

The death march to the next aid station was horrible. I tried eating one of the gels, but threw up immediately. I knew the low would continue until I ate something, but I was out of options. To make matters worse, sleep deprivation was beginning to set in and my slower-than-anticipated pace wasn't fast enough to keep me warm. I spent most of that section formulating how I was going to tell Shelly and Jesse I was done.

When I hobbled into the aid station, I started explaining how crappy I felt. I told them about the lack of food and the inability to eat gels without throwing up. I told them I was tired and sleepy. They silently nodded as they refilled my bottles and handed me some sort of hot soup. I didn't eat it as I started to explain that I wanted to quit.

They ignored me.

I repeated myself.

They finally stopped and looked at each other for a second. Shelly grabbed my arm and dragged me over to the campfire the aid station volunteers had made. She borrowed a blanket from a volunteer and instructed me to take a quick nap. I figured I'd try convincing them I was quitting after waking up.

I closed my eyes, but couldn't really sleep. I was wavering in that weird stage between states of consciousness—aware of my surroundings yet seemingly dreaming. Shelly and Jesse were standing about five feet from me discussing my situation. They weren't going to let me drop. A few minutes passed and they decided it was time for me to get moving. I vividly recall this conversation (with some moderate paraphrasing):

Jesse: "He needs to get moving to stay ahead of the cutoff; we should wake him up."

Shelly: "Let's poke him with a stick."

Jesse: "That's awesome! There's a pointy one."

There was a few second pause, then I felt a hard poke in the ribs. I didn't move. Another poke followed by giggling. I didn't move.

Shelly: "I bet he'll get up if I poke him in the butt."

It's worth noting that Shelly *never* bluffs. When we first started dating, I made a joke about her punching like a girl. She told me she was going to punch me in the nuts. I laughed. She punched me in the nuts. Hard.

Oh yeah, we were in a car on the highway and I was driving. *Shelly never bluffs.*

I mumble "I'm getting up" as I struggle to get my stiff, painful limbs to cooperate. Apparently it's not fast enough, because Shelly got one last poke . . . right between the cheeks.

To her credit, I *did* immediately jump up and was now wide awake. Thankfully I was feeling significantly better. They handed me another cup of soup, my water bottles, and flashlight, and shoved me toward the trailhead.

The next climb almost immediately after the aid station was long and fairly steep. I felt good for the first few minutes before I crashed again. I strongly considered turning around at that point, but figured Shelly and Jesse had already left to the next rendez-vous point. I continued on. The next ten to fifteen miles were pure hell. I don't think I ran a single step, instead opting for a zombie-like shuffle. I was cold, in pain, ridiculously sleepy, and wanted nothing more than to go home. I was cursing this damned sport. I knew I had to keep slogging along until I reached the turnaround point, which is where I'd see Jesse and Shelly again.

Sometime after daybreak I came to what I thought was the turnaround point. There were no other runner crews in sight, only volunteers. I talked to a teenage volunteer. I told him I wanted to drop, but needed to find my crew. I was sort of deliri-ous at that point, so my message probably didn't come out as smoothly as I thought it did. He pointed me up an asphalt road. I assumed the crews must be up there. I limped up the hill until I got to a parking lot on the summit. The only vehicle was an RV. A gentleman was standing by the door drinking a cup of coffee. I asked him where the crews were. He chuckled and told me they were past the aid station in the other direction. This climb was just another one of the turnarounds on the course. After I silently cursed the kid, I headed back down to the aid station. This time I talked to the aid station captain. I clearly told him I wanted to drop out of the race. He pointed down the road and told me my crew should be at the next intersection, but I had to make it to the actual turnaround point to give them my bib number.

Who knew quitting would be so damn hard!

I continued my unsteady walk down the road. I finally reached Jesse and Shelly about an hour later. Based on my time, they had assumed I walked the entire distance since they had seen me last. I simply said "I'm done." Shelly asked if I was sure, and

I was. They knew I had reached my breaking point. I still had to do the last out and back, but it was a little easier with company. We reached the aid station, I officially dropped, and we made the descent back to the Suburban. I had officially DNFed my second hundred-miler.

Grindstone was one of the most humbling experiences of my life. I went into it thinking I had mastered this sport only to get a severe ass-whooping. It made me question everything I had *supposedly* learned before. Was Western States just an incredible fluke? It was clear I made a slew of really stupid mistakes at Grindstone, but did I have the knowledge and skills to correct them in the future? Was there a piece of the puzzle that was missing? These were the questions that fueled my desire to try again. I cross-referenced our clinic schedule with the schedule of hundred-milers and found another great race: the Bighorn 100 in Sheridan, Wyoming. I would have about eight months to work out the kinks and do a lot more experimentation.

Our travels continued to provide us with ample opportunities to explore new mountain trails, chat with fellow ultrarunners, and work on my problem solving. We ran the Dallas White Rock Marathon, and I ran the Across the Years seventy-two-hour race, the Rodeo Valley and San Juan 50k races in California, and a few smaller road races. By the time the Pineland Farms fifty-miler came along at the end of May, I had already put in more training and racing miles than I had the entire previous year. I had gotten to the point where I could solve any problem that surfaced . . . except one.

At Across the Years, I had experienced what seemed sort of like dehydration. I tried fixing the problem by drinking plenty of water and electrolytes, but it didn't help. The only solution was to sit down and rest. The same phenomenon occurred on a Boulder-to-Nederland run with Jesse and one of his friends. I figured both incidents were a weird fluke so I ignored them.

When Bighorn came along, our schedule allowed Shelly and me to spend about eight weeks at altitude to acclimate for the mountain running in the Bighorn mountain range. This also gave us the opportunity to scout the trails. Shelly would be running the fifty-miler while I ran the hundred. My race started at 11 a.m., hers at 5 a.m. the following morning. My course was an out-and-back while her race started at the turnaround point. Both races would end at roughly the same time. It was a cool idea. I was running the race without a crew or pacer; instead relying on my drop bags and the aid stations.

The race started off as planned. It was a stunningly beautiful but difficult course. There were some monster climbs, rocky trails, and little cover from the sun. At night, the temperature dropped below freezing. Small problems popped up, but I managed to handle them competently. I avoided serious lows and enjoyed the highs. For most of the race I was on pace for about a twenty-seven or so hour finish, which was right about where I wanted to be.

The first signs of trouble hit on the first major climb during the morning of the second day. The temperature was increasing rapidly and I was beginning to sweat a lot. I started drinking a little more than normal to compensate. Within about thirty minutes I went from feeling great to absolutely terrible . . . and it was the exact same feeling I had at Across the Years and the Boulder-to-Ned run. Since I assumed it was dehydration, I started drinking even more along with the appropriate amount of electrolyte replacement. This strategy worked until I came to the more remote aid stations. They had to hike supplies several miles over rough terrain, so they only had a limited supply of water. Not wanting to take water from the runners behind me (which included the people running the fifty-miler), I only filled one bottle.

With somewhere around eighteen miles to go, conditions were deteriorating rapidly. I felt incredibly hot but didn't want to remove my tech shirt for fear of severe sunburn. I dunked my head in every little stream I crossed, then eventually started refilling my bottles with the untreated water. By the time I got to the last aid station with access to roads, I was ready to quit. Since I didn't have a crew, I would have to bum a ride off someone. Unfortunately I couldn't find anyone that was leaving, and one of the aid station volunteers told me they'd give me a ride . . . in about four hours. I made the decision to continue on.

The next sixteen miles were absolute hell, though not quite as bad as the original Burning River hell or the Grindstone "limp through the night" hell. Still, it was bad. The worst part of Bighorn is the end. Because it's a fairly large race, the finish line is held about two miles from the trailhead. Once the runners leave the trail, the remainder of the race is run on gravel and asphalt roads. I was *slowly* walking along the road when a car pulled up and Shelly jumped out. She had run into some trouble, DNFed, and got a ride back to the finish. She knew what time I had checked in at the aid stations and timed it perfectly. She walked me to the finish a few minutes over thirty-two hours, well above my earlier twenty-seven-hour pace.

After I had a few days to recover, I started researching the possible cause of the weird "crash" I experienced. I had suspected dehydration, but it didn't quite feel right (I've woken up dehydrated on quite a few occasions). I started connecting the dots. All of the events happened in hot, sunny, dry climates. All occurred after lengthy exposure to the elements. There was one variable that was still missing . . . what could it be? The epiphany happened when I saw a dog lying in the shade along a trail on a hot sunny day. *This* was the variable that was causing my problems.

What was that mystery variable?

Moisture-wicking technical T-shirts.

The idea is pretty simple. Sweat cools the body by evaporation. The moisture-wicking material moves sweat from the body so the evaporation takes place on the surface of the shirt. In humid weather, this isn't a factor because the shirt becomes saturated and the wet shirt still cools the body. However, hot dry weather causes the body to overheat due to a loss of evaporative cooling. The solution is simple, too, which I discussed in the "thermoregulation" section: *run shirtless.* Alternatively, run in cotton shirts that don't wick sweat easily.

SECTION 8:
THE RACE

PRERACE ROUTINE

Before the race begins, it's helpful to have a set routine. This allows you to prepare for the race without forgetting an important detail. You'll arrive at the starting line fully prepared. This routine can be practiced with training runs or shorter races. The practice allows you to tweak various variables.

My own routine developed over the years but always followed the same basic format. I would have all my clothes and gear laid out the night before and would set two alarms. I'm paranoid that way. When the alarms went off, I would drag myself out of bed, put in my contacts, and make coffee. I'd usually drop a deuce, drink some coffee, and fill my water bottles. I'd then check the local weather report for the day, take a second pipe-clearing deuce, and take a shower. Next came tape on the nipples and lubing all areas prone to chafing. I'd get dressed and carefully tie my shoes. Next I would double check my gear (bottles, flashlight batteries, a spork, etc.) and then head out to the race.

To establish timing for the routine, I would start with the start time and work backward. I liked to get to the start about forty-five minutes early, then add the commute time including parking. I had timed the hotel room routine repeatedly and could accomplish everything leisurely in about an hour. If Shelly was with me, we'd usually enjoy an "intimate session" to help relax. In that case, the hotel preparation took approximately an hour and thirty seconds.

LOSING WEIGHT FOR RACE DAY

Should you try to lose weight prior to race day? It depends. Generally speaking, the less you weigh, the more efficient you become. If you're at a healthy body weight, I would not recommend losing more. If you are overweight, trying to drop a few pounds might help you get to the finish line.

Due to my love of food and beer, I regularly pack on anywhere from fifteen to twenty-five extra pounds between races. As my goal races approach, I usually try to cut that down a bit. I've found my ideal race weight to be around 175 to 180 pounds (I'm six feet tall). I find the natural process of training usually takes care of the added weight. As my weekly running and cross-training increases, my caloric expenditure surpasses my caloric intake. If that doesn't work, I fall back on the greatest weight loss secret in the world: *I deliberately eat less and move more.* But I don't give up candy. Or beer.

Should you lose weight? I'd recommend a few simple tests:

For the guys: Strip down naked. Reach your arms above your head. Look down. Can you see your penis? Don't cheat—erections don't count. If you can, you're good. If you can't, you might consider losing a few pounds prior to the race.

For the ladies [from Shelly]: Designate a pair of your "A" pants. You know, the pants that you know make your ass look great. If they fit, you're right where you want to be. If they're tight, lose a few pounds.

RACE ETIQUETTE

There are a few unwritten rules of racing. Most runners learn these lessons by experience . . . mostly by inadvertently breaking the rules. This becomes a little more complicated because road races and trail races have slightly different etiquette. Here are the major trail race "rules":

- **Start in a position relative to your pace:** Trails are often congested at the beginning of trail races due to a large number of people funneling down relatively narrow trails. Start in a position relative to your ability. If you're fast, start near the front. If you're slow, start near the back. If you plan on walking at the start (not uncommon for hundred-milers), start at the very back.

- **Passing:** Passing rules are based on the commonly held trail traffic guidelines mentioned earlier in the book (tips from Mark Norfleet and Jacobus Degroot). Since trail races are commonly held on single track trails, passing etiquette is important. As a general rule, always pass on the left. Announce you're about to pass by saying "passing on the left." Thank the person you pass. Build good karma by wishing them luck.
- **Getting passed by a faster runner:** Always yield to someone faster. If someone approaches from behind and asks to pass, either step off to the right side of the trail or move as far right as possible. Again, wish him or her good luck.
- **On hills:** The person going uphill always has the right of way, so the person going down should yield and allow them to pass. However, I make an exception if the downhill runner is a faster runner. On an out-and-back course, it's common for a mid pack runner like me to meet the leaders as they're coming back from the turn around point. If I'm going up and they're coming down, I'll yield to them.
- **Non-racers:** If you encounter non-racers, the same trail rules apply. Always yield to vehicles, mounted animals, and pack animals. Mountain bikers are supposed to yield to runners, but be careful. In my experience, only about half of all mountain bikers actually follow that rule.
- **Littering:** Littering is not acceptable under any circumstance. In road races, it's common for runners to toss their cups, empty gel packets, or other crap on the ground after an aid station or along the course under the assumption that the race volunteers will clean up their mess. In trail races, this behavior is strictly forbidden. In

fact, some race directors are beginning to automatically disqualify those that litter. I applaud their efforts. Keep nature beautiful and don't expect volunteers to clean up after your sloppy ass.

- **Treat volunteers with the respect they deserve:** Volunteers are donating their time for *you*. Don't yell at them, berate them, or insult them. Not all volunteers will be experienced ultrarunners, so don't get upset if they make a mistake or can't fulfill your every request. When leaving an aid station, thank the volunteers for donating their time.

- **Don't complain:** This is a tough thing for some chronic complainers, but the rest of us would appreciate it. Don't complain about trivial matters like aid station food selection, volunteers, the race director, the difficulty of the course, weather, etc. Trail racing is supposed to be a challenge. If you're not up for the challenge and unpredictability of a trail race, stay at home.

- **Pooping:** If you have to drop a deuce during the race, move off the trail. The terrain usually determines the distance, but twenty feet should be considered a minimum. Also, try to get behind some sort of visual barrier. It's never cool to round a corner and catch a glimpse of someone pinching a loaf trail-side. On a semi related note, don't grab aid station food with the same hand used to wipe (tip from Jason Griffith).

- **Music:** Many runners prefer to listen to music while running. If you choose to listen to music, please have the decency to use headphones. I don't want to listen to Taylor Swift rant about the angst caused by a breakup she initiated at mile sixty of an ultra. If you are using headphones, keep the volume low so you can hear other runners trying to pass (tip from Kelsey Gray, Jocelyn Anderson, and Caleb Wilson). Alternatively, you can leave one ear bud out (tip from Vanessa Rodriguez).

- **Spitting and snot rockets:** If you have to spit or blow a snot rocket, make sure nobody is in the line of fire. Be sure you take the wind into account (tip from Louie Auslander).

- **Obstacles:** If you have to move a branch out of the way, don't let it snap back on the person immediately behind you (tip from Krista Cavendar). Also, warn people behind you of any major obstacle on the trail like deep holes, huge rocks, rattlesnakes, ill-placed dookie, etc. (tip from Caleb Wilson). Use your discretion, though. There's no need to blurt out every single irregularity.

- **Trail markings:** Trail markings are the objects used to mark a course. Since trail races are usually run in areas with multiple intersecting trails, the trail markings are necessary to keep runners on the right track. The most common materials used are ribbons, glow sticks (at night), signs, and ground markings. Different races use different markings depending on terrain, environment, and availability of volunteers to mark the course. It's important to attend prerace meetings and read course descriptions to determine how the course will be marked and what materials will be used.

In some cases, trail markings may be removed intentionally or unintentionally by other trail users. It's also possible for animals to eat the markings. At the Bighorn hundred-miler, it's not uncommon for elk to eat the ribbons used for marking.

When running any race, pay attention to markings instead of blindly following other runners. Race directors will usually give an approximate distance between markers. If you cover significantly more than that distance and don't see a marker, there's a good chance you went off course. Backtrack until you find the last marker, and then continue on from there.

THE RACE EXPERIENCE

If you've properly trained, the race shouldn't produce any surprises. You'll be ready for the inevitable highs and lows, the occasional boredom, the soreness, and the desire to quit. You'll be prepared to confront any problems that arise as soon as they appear. *Never ignore a problem, no matter how small.* The race should go smoothly and you'll love every second.

"Should" is the operative word in that last sentence. In a perfect world, every part of an ultra *should* be as enjoyable as riding a unicorn through a forest of Girl Scout Cookie trees.

Unfortunately that's never the case. Parts of the race are going to suck. You're going to experience fatigue and pain. You're going to be hungry, thirsty, and maybe nauseous. You'll develop blisters and chafe in places that seem impossible. You're going to get dirty, sweaty, and you're going to smell like an old gym shoe. You'll get too hot and too cold. You're going to obsess about the number of miles you have remaining. You're going to curse yourself for taking up this stupid hobby. You're going to plead with yourself to quit and go home.

When I started ultras, I was naive enough to believe I could simply will myself to continue if things went south. I've met one or two people that genuinely seem to have that ability, but the rest of us mortals will eventually crumble. If one or two things go wrong, it's not hard to power though. When five or six things go bad, we usually reach our limits. While you may be one of those "iron will" folks, it's safer to assume you're going to give up when the problems begin to compound. This is why it's important to solve problems *as soon as they appear.* When I was running Western States, I developed a small blister on my foot around mile eighty. I was feeling great and needed to maintain my pace to have any chance at finishing under twenty-four hours. The small blister didn't slow me down and was barely noticeable. However, I knew it would only continue to grow. I chose to stop, remove my shoe, lance the blister, fill the cavity with super glue, and relube the area. The entire process took around five precious minutes, but the problem was solved. Had I ignored it, the blister would have grown. I hit a low around mile ninety, and that blister pain could have been enough to cause me to DNF or slow down to the point where I wouldn't have met my time goal.

Expect problems to arise. Deal with the problems immediately. If it helps, use the mental checklist idea in the next section. This approach will help you deal with the psychological lows that can sabotage your race.

RUN-WALK STRATEGY

Walking during races? By now, you probably understand the necessity of walking. For ultrarunners, it's often a requirement to finish. For new runners, it's the preferred method to build endurance. For serious road runners, it's considered a mortal sin. But it's rarely something we practice.

Jeff Galloway has made a living coaching runners to use a run-walk strategy when racing . . . and it really works! The idea is simple: by interspersing walking breaks with periods of running, you can run faster and cut time off your finishes. Galloway has published a ton of books to help guide runners to the finish line using the run-walk-run method.

You don't necessarily need a book, though. I prefer to use the run-walk-run method based on feel. I run until I need a break, then walk until I feel recovered enough to run again. Then repeat.

I don't do this in training too often, but I *do* like to work on fast-walking skills. Since we see the walk break as a rest period, we tend to stroll along at a leisurely pace. Unfortunately, this wastes a lot of time. If we can cut our walking pace from twenty-minute miles down to around ten- to twelve-minute miles, we'll dramatically improve our finish times while still benefiting from the recovery periods afforded by the walk breaks. Much like speed training for running, speed training for walking will make your "cruising speed" more comfortable.

WALKING TECHNIQUE

Many people, especially barefoot and minimalist shoe runners, ask about walking technique. Do you land heel-toe or toe-heel? I alter my technique based on terrain. On flat, smooth terrain, I use the heel-toe technique with slightly longer steps. On rough terrain, I shorten my stride and use a toe-heel technique (much like I do when running).

Since walking produces only a fraction of the ground reaction force of running, use whatever technique feels most comfortable.

SPEEDING UP STRATEGY

The following section was a blog post I wrote about my initial experimentation with speeding up when tired. I had been doing mostly slow trail running, but was worried about a timed race on asphalt in the near future. Since this first experiment, I've successfully used the strategy in every ultra I've run.

This post was inspired by a thirty-four-mile training run with Jesse Scott. We were training for the Mind the Ducks :00 ultra in Rochester, New York. To help prepare us trail runners for half a day on asphalt, we decided to run on a paved bike path.

At about mile twenty, Jesse decided to mix things up a bit by adding the occasional "speed up." At a specific landmark, we'd essentially start sprinting until we reached another landmark. The distances varied from about fifty meters to one hundred meters or so. Our pace throughout the run was in the ballpark of 9–9:45 minute miles; the sprint pace was probably about 5:15 for Jesse and 6:40 for me. It was a good method to add interest to an otherwise tortuous run.

I noticed something else, too. Even though it was tough to initiate the sprint, the sprint itself felt shockingly *good*. After we slowed down, my muscles felt loose and free. I was able to cruise at a faster pace. My mood improved. I was shocked that I felt great, even after twenty-plus miles on roads. We ended up doing seven or eight of these "speed ups" in fairly rapid succession.

Between speed ups, we talked about the typical walking strategy used in ultras. Many runners will begin walking at a very early pace to conserve energy to perform better later in the race. I tried this strategy in my early ultra days but found it didn't work for me. I slowed my overall pace to the point where cutoffs became an issue. It also didn't seem to delay the point of extreme fatigue.

I found a more effective strategy was to run as long as I could, then add walk breaks when necessary. Note: I walk uphills the entire course for anything over a 50k. This resulted in a pretty good improvement in finish times.

I still had a problem, though. Once I started walking, the transition from running to walking and back would be painful. I didn't get much relief from walking, and it killed my pace once I started running again. In essence, walking made me feel *worse*.

After this last experiment with speed ups, I think I may try implementing this in my races. Instead of walking, I will try speeding up instead of taking walk breaks. I have to find the ideal ratio of speed ups. Jesse and I did one about every half mile, which was far too often. I may start at every two to three miles and observe the results. It defies conventional wisdom, but I've had a great deal of success doing the opposite of everybody else.

Logic seems to predict this idea will be an abysmal failure. It would seem as though the strategy would be excessively taxing on your body. Or would it? From a physiological standpoint, I can't hypothesize what effects this has. Would the net effects be better or worse?

My optimism toward this strategy stems from seeing it in action. The strategy has worked very well for Jesse. During the Woodstock fifty-miler, he dramatically sped up whenever he hit gravel roads. He won the race by about an hour. I also cannot deny the effect it had on our run. I felt *much* better after our speedup than after stopping to eat.

MENTAL CHECKLIST

I like to think of ultras as puzzles. Each race is a set of problems that must be solved. Training teaches me how to anticipate and correctly diagnose the problems, then devise solutions based on my limited resources. Some are obvious. If I trip and fall or get attacked by a mountain lion, "broken limb" or "severe cougar bites" won't go unnoticed. Otherwise, it's surprisingly easy to ignore or miss problems when they first appear. Sometimes I get lost in my own thoughts, get distracted by the scenery, or I'm conversing with other runners. I developed a routine to combat this problem. About every fifteen minutes during races, I'll go through a mental checklist as a means of monitoring my physical and psychological state. This is a sample of the questions I ask myself:

- Am I eating enough?
- Am I showing any warning signs of entering a "low," which is usually indicated by depressing thoughts?

- When is the last time I urinated?
- What color was the urine?
- Are any muscles cramping?
- Is the temperature rising or falling?
- Am I dressed appropriately to maintain body temperature?
- Am I chafing?
- Am I developing hot spots on my feet?
- Is my pace too fast or too slow?

If I detect a problem, I solve it immediately. Small problems grow to huge problems quickly. If I can't solve the problem out on the trail, I'll take care of it at the next aid station.

SHAVE THE JUNK OR ROCK THE 'FRO?

This is probably more of an issue for dudes, and wouldn't even be considered if it weren't for the "metrosexual manscaping" movement of the late 1990s and early 2000s.

Here's my "too much information" story. Around the time I started running ultras, I also started experimenting with various methods of trimming. It was done purely for aesthetics (Shelly liked it). I was surprised to find two effects: the trimming seemed to keep the groin region cooler and it dramatically reduced chafing. Seeing the positive effects of cutting back the schlong-fro, I decided to try shaving. As expected, the results were even better. Since that time, I've continued a routine of shaving.

A few tips and points to consider before giving your boys the Bruce Willis 'do:

- **When the hair starts to grow back, it's itchy as hell for a few days.** You have to either endure the discomfort or keep shaving at least once a week.
- **If trimming, don't use the closest setting on electric clippers.** Loose skin can get caught between the blades. Yes, it hurts. A lot.
- **If shaving, it's much easier to trim first.** Long hair is difficult to shave. I use the trimmer to shorten the hair, then bust out the razor.
- **Pleasure.** Not to turn this into a sex manual or anything, but the skin-on-skin clitoral contact may be pleasurable for women.

I do feel compelled to offer a warning. You may decide to channel the 1970s and let the bush go. You may also figure out that a blow dryer is effective at drying the nether region. If you're ever caught in the act by your significant other, don't answer the "What are you doing?!?" question with "Warming dinner!"

On a closely related topic, I occasionally get questions about . . . butt hair. We're not talking about the hair toward the outside of the cheeks; more like the hair *in the crack*. Earlier, I mentioned the possibility of butt-crack chafing, and the remote possibility of the cheeks fusing together as they heal. The handful of brave souls that have volunteered accounts of their experiences reveal a mixed bag. Ass hair may help prevent chafing, or it may help promote *worse* chafing. Since individual results vary, I would add it to the list of variables to test in training.

CAFFEINE

Caffeine is the world's most popular psychoactive drug . . . and the secret to many ultra finishes. For ultrarunning purposes, caffeine is useful because it can decrease fatigue, increase mental alertness, and ward off sleep. It's also a mild pain reliever, which is the reason it's included in many over-the-counter pain medications. Sounds pretty good, right?

For ultras, caffeine can be incredibly useful when used properly. When shit's about to go bad, caffeine can save the day. I use it mostly during the very early morning hours of hundred-milers in the form of coffee during cold weather and either Red Bull or Monster (both energy drinks) in warmer weather. All provide a near-instant boost with little negative side effects.

Caffeine issues aren't without controversy or potential dangers. First, caffeine is a mild diuretic. It makes you pee more than normal, which can lead to dehydration. I solve this problem by only using caffeine if I'm well hydrated. Second, it is possible to overdose on caffeine. At the very least, too much caffeine will cause profuse sweating, tremors, and hallucinations . . . all of which would suck during an ultra. Finally, caffeine increases heart rate. If you have heart issues, this could also be fatal. The rapid heart rate may also interfere with efficiency by wearing you out faster.

I solve all of these problems through prerace experimentation. I know exactly how much caffeine I can consume over a given amount of time. Waiting until I absolutely need the boost eliminates a lot of the dehydration problems. Using it in moderation limits the dangers due to overdose and the "crash" after the effects wear off. Currently, that limit is two servings of energy drinks throughout an entire hundred-mile race, one about three hours after the first. Logistically, this usually means one at 2 a.m. and another at 5 a.m.

Testing caffeine use can be a bit tricky since the conditions in training should match the conditions you'll experience in a race. The best test would be during long overnight runs. If that's not possible, simply staying up all night, á la a preteen slumber party, can be an adequate substitute. Try different forms of caffeine. Consider palatability, ability to pack in drop bags, or if it can be carried with you. Coffee, tea, energy drinks, caffeine pills, energy gum, and soda are all possibilities. You'll likely find one delivery method to be more effective than others.

ELECTROLYTES

Back when I started running ultras, the consumption of supplemental electrolytes was more or less a given. If you were running long, you needed to be consuming a product like S! Caps, Salt Sticks, or good ole rock salt. The logic made sense—you had to replace the salt lost via sweat. When combined with water consumption, runners risked hyponatremia.

I would take one S! Cap about every hour or so depending on temperature. My sweat would get saltier and saltier, which led to burning eyes and chafing (salt deposits around the groin and armpits is much like having sex on a beach—grit + friction = unpleasant results).

Of course, the electrolytes *did* dramatically reduce the danger of hyponatremia. The problem had more to do with an overconsumption of water, and the electrolyte overconsumption was an unfortunate side effect. I had a lot of friends that read Tim Noaks's book *Waterlogged*. I haven't read it myself, but their ad nauseum discussions pretty much summed up the plot: *drink to thirst.*

I started following this advice, first at the 2012 Grand Mesa hundred-miler, then the 2012 TransRockies six-day stage race, and lastly at the 2012 Grindstone hundred-miler. In all three races, I cut my water consumption considerably . . . with no ill effects. The other benefit: I didn't require any electrolyte supplementation. I did get some electrolytes from the various gels I ate, along with the half pound of bacon I ate ten hours before the race. Aside from that, I was electrolyte-free. The result: my sweat was not especially salty. At Grindstone, I didn't have any salt-induced chafing issues. As long as I didn't overdrink, I had no need to supplement electrolytes.

But what about symptoms like cramping?

As I discussed in the section earlier, many in the ultrarunning community seem to believe hot temperatures can be remedied by drinking more water and taking more electrolytes. Unfortunately, the body only has a finite ability to cool itself via sweat (and moisture-wicking materials may dramatically reduce that ability). So . . . the solution isn't necessarily drinking more liquid and popping more salt. The solution could be taking steps to cool down. Here are a few:

- **Slow down.** Movement generates heat. More movement generates more heat. To cool down, slow down.
- **Seek shade.** No explanation needed.
- **Ditch clothes.** Unless the clothing is intended to reflect heat (white clothing in the desert) or act as a solar furnace, less is more. If that means running naked, so be it. We're all beautiful . . . might as well show off your goods.
- **Get wet.** Dousing yourself with water facilitates evaporative cooling. Cooler water also helps cool the body (via conduction).
- **Expose yourself to a breeze.** This also helps facilitate evaporative cooling (via convection).

Reframing the problem from hydration/electrolyte imbalance to thermoregulation has resulted in great success for me personally. I also have quite a few friends that have toyed around with these ideas and experienced similar positive results.

UPSET STOMACH

Nausea is a pretty common condition during ultras. Digestively speaking, bad things happen when mixing extreme exercise and ingesting junk food. It's not unusual to see pools of vomit along the trail. With experience, you'll eventually develop the ability to identify a variety of partially digested snack foods.

"Looks this runner really loved his Oreos, potato chips, and turkey sandwiches."

I've never had much of a problem with an upset stomach during races due to my continuous gluttony training, but I've prepared nonetheless. It's rare that I get an upset stomach, so training for the condition has always proved difficult. My solution? I waited until I contracted the stomach flu, then did a long run.

First, this was a terrible idea. Experimenting can be fun, but contending with chills, body aches, and nausea while running was one of the worst experiences of my life. The fact that it was winter in Michigan made it even worse.

Second, I did manage to glean some useful methods of alleviating nausea. The standard treatments during races usually consist of, in order of popularity, cola, Tums, crackers or bread, ginger candies, and Pepto-Bismol. I tried each one in about forty-five- to sixty-minute intervals. Cola and Tums helped. Pepto-Bismol, bread, and crackers didn't seem to produce any effect. Ginger candies? Unfortunately I tried those last after eating everything else. Not only did ginger candies not help, the flavor caused me to gag and projectile vomit everything else I had consumed. The pinkish-brown bread vomit frozen to my coat really completed the experience.

DIARRHEA

I may have been stupid enough to experiment with nausea, but I'm not brave enough to intentionally run while experiencing diarrhea. Early in my ultra career, I never experienced diarrhea during a training run or a race. Still, it always scared the shit out of me.

Okay, that may be the worst joke in the book.

Anyway, I heard enough horror stories from experienced ultrarunners to know diarrhea was almost always a game ender. Not only would it lead to dehydration, but the time spent squatting off the trail would usually place you in danger of missing cutoff times. The frequent wiping and/or less-than-thorough wiping could cause ass chafing. We won't even discuss the catastrophic "I shit my pants" scenarios.

The sheer terror of the worst-case diarrhea scenarios compelled me to carry two Immodium pills during most long runs and all races. If it was going to happen, I'd be prepared, damn it!

Eventually, it did happen. The year was 2011. We made a road trip from Michigan to New York to run the second annual Mind the Ducks twelve-hour race in Rochester, New York. It's the same race I mentioned earlier in the book. The course consisted of a half-mile asphalt loop around a pond. The goal was to finish as many laps as possible.

I began feeling under the weather two days before the event. Like most ultrarunners, I ignored the symptoms. I woke up the next morning feeling pretty terrible. I powered through it and continued eating as I would before any race. I had a running clinic that afternoon at a local Crossfit gym. I'd like to say it went well, but I honestly don't remember anything. I had a fever and seemed to be hallucinating. Before bed, I tried my favorite homeopathic flu cure: beer and spicy chicken wings. I was sleeping by 7 p.m.

Sidebar: Never follow my homeopathic health advice.

I felt pretty good the next morning . . . for about five minutes. I was still feverish, still seemed to be hallucinating a bit, and was experiencing stomach cramps. I somehow managed to go through the motions of my prerace routine. Within an hour, we were at the course preparing for the start. According to Shelly, I looked like death warmed over. I convinced myself the cure was running the race even though it hurt to walk from the car to the event tent.

As I was signing in, the girl at the table recognized me. At that point, my barefoot book had been doing well, I had written for a few national publications, and I had appeared on a few regional and national TV and radio shows. I was sort of famous among a tiny niche group within the running community. It was my one and only "I'm a huge fan and am speechless" interaction. Unfortunately I was delirious to the point where I didn't really understand what was going on. Shelly, who was standing next to me, recounted the story. Apparently I just mumbled a thank you and stumbled away. She teased me about the interaction for years.

Once the race actually started, I felt better . . . for about an hour. I was slow but made good progress. As time went on, I thought the illness seemed to be lifting. I was beginning to enjoy the race. Our crew was doing well. Jesse Scott went on to win the race, Shelly ran well, Mark Robillard set a distance PR, and our non-runner friend John DeVries amassed around twenty-two miles with zero training. Things were looking up . . . until the diarrhea hit.

Luckily, the loop was only a half mile and there were two Porta-Potties. The first "incident" came on suddenly. I spent about five minutes relieving myself of the liquid Satan that occupied my bowels, all the while regretting my spicy food decision the day before. Once I finished, I felt significantly better. I got back out on the course and started running.

For one lap.

As I rounded the last corner before the Porta-Potties, the urge returned. Back to the Porta-Potties. After a few more minutes on the toilet, I stopped at my gear bag and popped two Immodium pills. I was certain the pipes were clean, so I went out for another lap. Things went well . . . for about half of the lap. Back to the Porta-Potties.

This "run a lap, then poop" pattern went on for what should have been a physiologically impossible period of time. The laps eventually devolved into a slow walk as the jostling made matters worse. The chafing from wiping eventually set in. This pattern continued for hours. I was determined to continue on for reasons I don't quite understand. The end finally came when John convinced me to mix tequila with the Heed sports drink in my water bottle. I earned a valuable lesson on that next lap: don't drink tequila during a race!

I finally threw in the towel after the loop. Thankfully, the explosive diarrhea ceased as soon as I stopped running. John, who also decided to throw in the towel, convinced me to make a beer run. We spent the final hours of the race cheering on the rest of our crew and thanking Shelley Viggiano, the ace director, for stocking ample toilet paper.

CHAFING

Chafing is a significant problem in ultras. The longer you run, the more likely you are to chafe. Any place where anything comes in contact with skin, including other skin, is susceptible to chafing. Your long runs will give you ample opportunity to learn what areas chafe and how they chafe, allowing you to experiment with solutions.

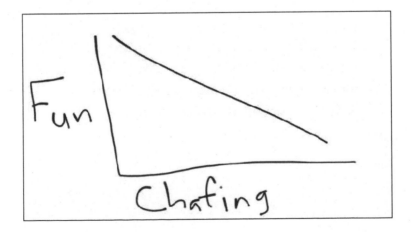

Here are my suggestions for various areas:

- **Nipples:** Cover with adhesive bandages. I used to use duct tape, but the adhesive irritated the skin after long hours of exposure. For added protection, add a dab of your favorite sports lube to the nipple prior to applying the bandage.
- **Groin/thighs:** I've tried quite a few options: various lubes, tape, compression shorts, a kilt (added ventilation), and various states of trimming and/or shaving. I finally found short running shorts (current favorite = Brooks Infinity III) and a liberal dose of SportSlick brand lube work wonders.
- **Armpits:** The 'pits are difficult to protect. The only real option I found was good ole lube.
- **Any area the clothing touches, including sports bras for the ladies:** Different articles of clothing will cause different levels of chafing. I prefer cotton shirts to technical shirts for this reason—the cotton is less abrasive. I usually treat trouble areas with a dab of lube or periodically change to a different style of clothing.
- **Hands (due to carrying water bottles):** My knuckles usually become chafed in long races. In cool weather, I've found fingered or fingerless gloves to be effective. In hot weather, I just lube up the knuckles.

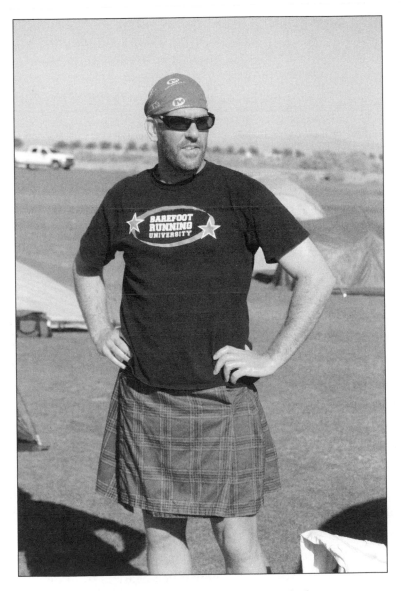

The kilt kept the undercarriage chafe-free.

AFTER THE RACE

Immediately after finishing a race, expect to be sore and stiff. These symptoms lessen with experience but can be quite dramatic for the first few races. After my first hundred-mile finish, I sat in a chair to enjoy a celebratory beer and hot dog. Fifteen minutes later, I couldn't stand up without help. It will take a few days to regain decent mobility. Plan to take the elevator. If you own a car with a manual transmission, you may want to hire a chauffeur.

Insomnia and night sweats are also common the night after a race. The extreme physical exertion really messes with circadian cycles and thermoregulation. For all of my races, I would wake up in the middle of the night drenched in sweat and unable to fall asleep. Eventually I started sleeping on towels.

Physical recovery from ultras takes some time. While our bodies are more than capable of phenomenal endurance feats, they do need to heal. Exactly how much changes from one individual to the next, and also changes as a function of experience. A common axiom in the running world suggests taking one day of recovery for every mile run. This is okay for a 5k (three days off) or even a half marathon (thirteen days off), but a fifty-miler? Taking almost two months off, unless injured, is ridiculous. Toss that axiom out the window.

In my own early ultra experiences, a fifty-miler would sideline me from running for at least a month. It would take several days before I could ascend or descent stairs, and maybe a week before I could walk with a relatively normal gait.

As my body adapted over the course of a few years, recovery time shrank. My last hundred-miler (Grindstone) wasn't too bad. I was able to run slowly the very next day. I felt normal after about three days. I was able to get back to ultra distances within about ten days.

When first beginning, take recovery slow. Get to know how your body responds. You'll be much more susceptible to injury and illness during the recovery period. I would recommend two weeks with little or no running and a month before getting back to normal training as a decent baseline until you get to know how your body responds.

POST-RACE DEPRESSION

In the weeks after your first few ultras, it's not uncommon to experience a temporary bout of depression. You've spent many months chasing a goal. The elation of finishing wears off. You're still in recovery mode and cannot get back to regular training. It's a weird phenomenon that seems to be almost universal. So how do you deal with it?

I found setting new goals and utilizing "active recovery" helped mitigate the post-race funk. I would find a new race and start developing a training plan that included very light recovery activities like walking, slow running, or swimming. The renewed focus helps alleviate the "lost" feelings.

Since some of the depressive symptoms could be physiological in nature (serotonin deficit?), I also change up my routine to utilize some self-help strategies. I eliminate as many stressors as I can and engage in more relaxing activities. I spend more time in the sun. If it's perpetually cloudy, which was common in West Michigan, I visit a tanning booth. I increase my consumption of spicy foods, which produce natural endorphines. All of these steps help me survive the unpleasant post-race depression. If you start developing severe symptoms (complete lack of motivation, profound sadness or hopelessness, suicidal thoughts, etc.) do not hesitate to seek professional help.

OBTAINING SPONSORSHIP

Occasionally people ask me about sponsorship because they assume I was a sponsored runner based on my representation of Merrell. Technically, I was a consultant and ambassador, which was a little different. I was paid to teach people how to run, not necessarily represent the brand during races. I wore Merrell shoes because they fit my particular feet perfectly. I did, however, get a lot of opportunities to work with various marketing departments from quite a few outdoor brands. That exposure gave me some interesting insight to the decision-making process brands use to determine which athletes (or events) they are going to sponsor.

The very short answer: brands sponsor athletes because they want to sell more products.

A slightly longer answer: a brand will sponsor anyone if it will result in a positive return on their investment. Nike was willing to pay Michael Jordan and Tiger Woods millions and millions of dollars because they were insanely popular athletes that resulted in huge sales.

Many runners erroneously believe the best way to obtain sponsorship is to win. That's an excellent start, but a winning athlete also needs a dedicated following to be able to help sell the company's product. The bigger the athlete's audience, the more value he or she has as a sponsor. I was a good brand ambassador because I had a dedicated blog following, had sold quite a few books, and was a veteran teacher, *not* because I was a great runner (I'm mediocre at best).

Dean Karnazes is a great example of this idea. Dean's a great runner, but certainly not the best ultrarunner in the world. Despite this, he has great value as a sponsored athlete because he's done a ton of really cool "publicity runs," has written some great books, and spends a lot of time traveling and interacting with his fans.

If you want to be a sponsored runner, you need to be doing something beyond running. You need to build an audience in some way. Writing books, directing races, holding clinics, producing podcasts, blogging, creating and maintaining social media groups, creating running groups, and producing instructional videos are all ways you can build an audience. It's an endeavor that takes a long time.

Once you have an audience, start approaching companies. Generally speaking, it's easier to obtain sponsorship from smaller local companies than gigantic international corporations. Use your Google searching skills to identify individuals in their marketing departments. Some companies make this easier by supplying sponsorship applications on their websites. Be warned: that's usually a sign they get *a lot* of applications and competition will be stiff. Mention anything that will give them a *snapshot of your audience*, not just your accomplishments.

Keep your expectations low. At the time of writing, trail running and ultrarunning are small niche markets. There's not a lot of money to be made from sponsorships. Even the most marketable runners barely make enough money to cover race entry fees and travel expenses. They usually get free gear. It's certainly not enough to make a living. As the sport grows this may change but is unlikely in the coming years.

SOLVING THE ULTRA PUZZLE

Bighorn had went exceptionally well . . . until it didn't. I was hoping it would be a redemption, the race that would prove to me that Western States wasn't a fluke. I ran into a serious problem that initially appeared to be dehydration. After some research, I deduced that it could be hyperthermia, or an increase in body temperature. Our travels took us from the Bighorn Mountains of Wyoming to Truckee, California, near Lake Tahoe (and Squaw Valley, the start of Western States). The hot, sunny, dry weather would be a perfect testing ground to test the theory.

To conduct the experiments, I would do long runs shirtless, wearing a moisture-wicking shirt, and a cotton shirt, track how much I drank before and during the run, and record my body temperature. After about a week, I noticed a small effect. My body temperature would increase when wearing the moisture-wicking shirt, but only if it was hot and dry enough for the shirt to remain dry due to rapid evaporation. If humidity was high and sweat saturated the shirt, my body temperature remained the same. The same thing happened if I regularly doused the shirt with water.

Armed with this knowledge, I was ready for our next running adventures. It started when Shelly and I joined friends Jon Sanregret and Krista Cavender to crew and pace Jesse Scott for the Tahoe Rim 100. In typical fashion, we drank too much the night before the race, then spent the next day and a half acting like juveniles. I paced Jesse for the final quarter of the race, which included the cold of the night and the building heat of the following day. Jesse finished well before the hottest part of the day, but the cotton shirt I wore seemed to work well.

This race was also where we attempted to start a new trend in the ultrarunning community. When spectators see a struggling runner, they increase their morale by flashing. The early returns on the positive effects of the practice are favorable.

After Jesse's Tahoe finish, we moved to Grand Junction, Colorado, to run the Grand Mesa 100. Shelly had DNFed the Javalina 100 earlier that year and was eager to try another hundo. Grand Mesa was known as a small "low key" ultra. There was very little fanfare, very basic support, and a small number of runners.

The most notable feature of the course was the descent off the mesa, then back up. Based on the elevation chart, we affectionately dubbed the race "The Devil's Vagina." Shelly and I planned to run the race together, and were joined by Jesse. Grand Mesa was only two weeks after Tahoe Rim, so his plan was to keep us company as long as possible.

The race went pretty well until we got to the bottom of the vagina . . . er, until we reached the aid station at the base of the mesa. Shelly and I (Jesse dropped at about mile forty) started the climb back to the top of the mesa as the sun was setting. We knew the climb was going to be difficult, so we decided to leave our second layer of warmer clothing in our drop bags. Things started going south when I led us off the trail and we wandered around for a mile or so. Eventually we made it back to the trail, but the climb was more difficult than we had anticipated. We were treated to a spectacular lightning show miles away. We were at about cloud level, which created an amazing light show. Hours later, we made it to the top. And it sucked. We were sleepy, exhausted, and hungry. The cold wind blowing across the open fields was too much. We stumbled down the asphalt road to the aid station at about mile sixty, occasionally stopping to lie on the still-warm blacktop in an attempt to stay somewhat warm. It felt as though we had wandered forever before a volunteer pulled up in a cargo van. He stopped to check on us, so we hitched a ride to the next aid station to formally DNF. He then gave us a ride to the start line.

The top of the mesa had reminded me of my hometown in rural northern Michigan, minus the altitude. There were lots of fields, cows, trees, and rolling hills. The scene was complete when we came across an overturned pickup truck. Our savior, the van driver, stopped to investigate. The driver was nowhere to be found and there were empty beer cans everywhere. The scene brought me back to my youth.

After Grand Mesa, we returned to Michigan to visit family as Shelly and I prepared for our next running adventure: the TransRockies-six day, hundred-twenty-five-mile stage race run through the mountains of Colorado. I had known of the race for a few years, but didn't consider it until our friends Vanessa and Shacky (Robert Shackleford) planned on running it. It was much more expensive than the most expensive ultras we had run, mostly due to the logistics. We camped each night between the stages and the race directors moved the entire camp from one location to the next. By that time, I had decided on my next hundred-mile test: I was going back to Grindstone.

TransRockies turned out to be an awesome experience, though the atmosphere and actual running was much different than a typical ultra. The event felt like a runner fantasy camp because we were continually pampered. The food was fantastic, the support was amazing, and the organizers catered to our every need. The vast majority of the runners camped in tents. This was one of my favorite parts of the experience as it built camaraderie. The only drawback was the silence. Shelly and I had a prerun routine we had to maintain. Despite our effort to be even quieter than we had to be in the RV, I'm sure some of our neighbors heard more than they bargained for. Camping sex is in tents.

The actual running was tough, but the course consisted of too much road running for my taste. The variety of conditions was an excellent opportunity to continue experimentation. I learned some valuable lessons. One morning I ate about twenty slices of bacon, which resulted in incredibly salty sweat. That led to severe groin chafing, which required some creative taping along the trail. Evidently many of the runners that passed weren't familiar with the lack of modesty that's common in ultras. In retrospect, I probably should have went a little farther off the trail to tape my junk. By the end, I knew I was ready for Grindstone.

Before leaving Michigan, we attended the Woodstock Trail Running Festival in Hell, Michigan. This was the site of the Hallucination 100, my first hundred-mile finish. The party-like hippy-themed atmosphere turned out to be a perfect storm for our "we don't take running seriously" shenanigans. If you are a serious runner that frowns on excessive drinking and engaging in frat party–like activities, it's probably better to skip ahead a few paragraphs.

We met up with a bunch of friends, including Jesse Scott and Christian and Amy Peterson. Our plan was to hang out, drink, and run some of the shorter races. We arrived the day before everyone else showed up. Christian convinced us to play a dumb drinking game called "wise wizards" where we duct taped our empty beer cans together end to end to create a wizard staff. The person with the longest staff won. I'm pretty sure we all lost the game that night. By the end of the evening we went skinny dipping in the pool and were running laps around the almost-empty campground naked.

The next day didn't get much better. We started drinking around 10 a.m. Admittedly this day was a bit of a blur. Lots of runners were arriving, so we chatted with a lot of our Michigan runner friends we hadn't seen in a long time. As evening approached, Randy Step, the race director, asked Shelly and me if we were interested in volunteering to help with the aid station at the 5k that night. It's a clothing-optional run. Apparently we had developed a reputation from our skinny dipping and naked laps the night before. We agreed.

The 5k was really cool. Being surrounded by people that aren't freaked out by nudity was a relatively new experience and *very* liberating. We had been drinking for around ten hours at that point and were considerably more intoxicated than everyone else. It didn't help that the aid station was serving alcohol. Almost everyone was super cool, though a few of the more serious runners seemed to be offended when Shelly started requesting naked chest bumps. We returned to the campsite and continued chatting until the wee hours of the morning.

The following day, Shelly, Christian, Jesse, and I all ran races. I had signed up for the half marathon because I needed a rest from the long runs. Jesse joined me for the shorter race. Shelly and Christian ran the 50k. I foolishly decided to run in "costume," which consisted of a tie-dyed tank top and scandalously short cutoffs. The lesson I learned: *Don't run in short cutoffs!* The chafing was significantly worse than the chafing I experienced after eating the pounds of bacon at TransRockies. Around mile eight I started experiencing pain in my right foot. The race proved to be more difficult than a cross-eyed teacher trying to control his pupils. Not wanting to risk further injury, I DNFed at mile ten.

Yes, I DNFed a half marathon. It was a low point of my running career. It wouldn't have mattered much anyway because I was about as hungover as I've ever been. Both Shelly and Christian also dropped from their respective races. The allure of continuing our partying was too great. Of the four of us, Jesse was the only one to finish. We spent the rest of the day hanging out, drinking, and congratulating the ultra finishers.

In retrospect, Woodstock signified an important shift. Over the last year or so, I wasn't running for the sake of running. Running had become a means of exploring mountain trails *or* an excuse to hang out with friends. I wasn't taking running nearly as seriously as I had in years past. I had always tried to keep the sport fun, but my book, blogging and freelance writing, and clinics had raised my profile enough where serious runners wanted me to be the voice of barefoot and minimalist shoe running. I was more than happy to share my experiences and teach, but I was acutely aware of the lack of actual research on the topic. I was also increasingly surrounded by people that were less concerned about the journey of running and more concerned about the tangible extrinsic rewards. It was becoming more and more difficult to have Woodstock-like experiences.

I was still focused on Grindstone, though. I needed to find out if my experimentation had paid off. I was about as prepared as I could possibly be. I had done a ton of other races and training runs over the last year. I had perfected nutrition and hydration, found good shoes, and had figured out the thermoregulation stuff. I was familiar with the course. I had gotten to a point where I was comfortable solving my own problems, so Shelly was my lone crew member and pacer. We spent a few weeks in Virginia before the race so we could train on the actual course.

The race went exactly as planned. I started conservatively, focused on enjoying the experience, and tackled the minor problems before they became major problems. There were no major surprises, though interesting things did happen. I came across a huge rattlesnake crossing the trail in the middle of the night. I heard what sounded like a woman screaming about a quarter of a mile off the trail in the middle of the night (which very well could have been a hallucination). Shelly paced me for the last thirty miles or so, which was a welcome distraction. I only experienced one significant low around mile ninety or so, but was able to mitigate the effects by eating before it really started. I ended up finishing a few minutes over twenty-nine hours, which was about nine hours under the cutoff. For me, the race was a resounding success. My finish time was significantly slower than Western States, but I felt great and didn't have a major problem I couldn't solve. After years of running ultras, I finally felt as though I had more or less figured them out.

After Grindstone, we traveled west. Shelly took another stab at a hundred-miler at Punkin Holler in Oklahoma, then we continued to Southern California. The last race I had on my schedule was another tough hundo, Steve Harvey's Chimera 100. Try as I might, I couldn't muster the motivation to prepare. The fire that had preceded every other race just wasn't there. Two days before, I still hadn't looked at a course map, packed my drop bags, or even figured out where the race was being held. About an hour before we were supposed to leave for the prerace meeting, I told Shelly I couldn't run. I had DNFed quite a few races over the years; this was my first *DNS*. Since Stephanie had planned on watching our kids for the weekend, we decided to get a hotel room and just relax. While my peers were running up and down the mountain trails of Chimera, we were eating Mexican food, drinking box wine, and watching reruns of *How I Met Your Mother*.

I expected to to feel guilty for missing the race, but I didn't. I felt relieved. I had fully immersed myself in the running world for years, had run somewhere around fifty races, written two or three books and close to a thousand blog posts, and held well over one hundred clinics. I was mentally and physically exhausted. I needed a break.

Shelly and I continued to run a few days each week. The San Diego area, where we decided to settle down for awhile, provided ample trails. Eventually we decided to sign up for another race and chose the San Diego Trail Marathon put on by Paul Jesse. It was a well-organized fun race, but we just weren't into it. At the time, I was challenging people to do silly stuff that helped over-come fear via my "BRUcrew" Facebook group (like do twenty pushups in the produce department of the local grocery store or hand out roses to random strangers on the street). Fear, after all, is nothing more than your brain telling you "This is going to be fucking epic!" One challenge was to DNF a race at the finish line. I chose this race. When we got to the finish, I had to explain to Paul that I was DNFing three feet before crossing the finish line. He laughed at my dumbass explanation. The other more seri-ous runners that had congregated at the finish weren't quite as understanding. I just shrugged.

At the time of writing, that last trail marathon was exactly one year ago. We're still hanging out in San Diego (the weather is far better than Michigan) and the laid-backedness agrees with our personalities. We put the nomad lifestyle on hold because it became too much of a grind. We craved a degree of stability. Besides, all the turnpikes were taking a toll.

Always one to try new stuff first, Shelly started training at the San Diego Fight Club, a local MMA gym run by former King of the Cage world champion and Brazilian jiujitsu black belt Charlie Kohler. After her second jiujitsu class, she easily choked me out while wrestling around. I signed up the next week. Over the last year, I've been focusing on jiujitsu, boxing, and kickboxing. Running got to a point where significant improvement would take more time and effort than I was willing to expend. I had reached a point of mastery, run enough races, and explored enough amazing mountain trails to sufficiently satisfy my curiosity. Improving times or running the same races over and over just doesn't satisfy me as much as exploration. Running no longer *scared* me. It was time for a new challenge, and the *possibility* of fighting in an MMA fight, especially as a thirty-eight-year-old dude, was just the challenge I needed. One of the first days I sparred, I faced a badass dude nicknamed "The Urinal." He didn't take any shit.

The time away from the sport has given me an opportunity to seriously reflect on the entirety of the experience. Before I started running, I was a seriously overweight mediocre football coach destined to toil away in a career that began to feel more like a prison sentence. In the decade since, I've underwent profound changes. I came to the realization that we only have a limited time before we die. Odds are good we have even less time to do something physically active. I also realized many of the limitations we place on ourselves (or allow others to place on us) are ridiculous. That led me to actively embrace that which I feared. Initially that was manifested by running the first fifty-miler, then the barefoot ultra, then a hundred-miler. Later it led me to self-publish a book despite nearly zero training as a professional writer. That led to two more self-published books, acquiring a literary agent, and publishing a book with a traditional publisher (this book is my second). I became a social media expert of sorts, learned a bachelor's degree—worth of exercise and physiology knowledge, and was able to become a "professional" nomadic runner. I've met thousands of awesome people, traveled to almost every state and three countries, and had the opportunity to spend significant time with my children. Running has also helped me control the occasional bout of acute depression brought on by stress or lack of sunlight (West Michigan is almost as cloudy as Seattle). I would have never imagined any of this would have been possible . . . until I started to do it.

For me, running wasn't necessarily the cause of the adventures I listed above. Running was the conduit that I used to explore. Running didn't necessarily change my life, but it did help me realize I had far more potential than I previously thought. It taught me that life should be enjoyed. Going through the motions in hopes of a payoff down the road is a sucker's bet. I have to enjoy today. If I have something I want to do before I die, I have to start doing it immediately.

Running also connected me with people that did play a pivotal role in changing my life. There are thousands of people that played small roles in every accomplishment I've done, and scores of people that have played major roles. Writing about my own running experiences is more of a celebration of the gratitude I feel toward those folks than a self-congratulatory pat on the back.

For some, though, running really *is* life changing. I've met hundreds of people that have used running to overcome obesity, drug addiction, or their own self-imposed limits that have resulted in chronic unhappiness. The effects seem amplified when combined with the serenity of trail running and the sheer difficulty of ultramarathons.

The purpose of this book is to convince you that pretty much anyone can be a trail runner and eventually tackle ultramarathons. All that's required is a desire and a willingness to put in the time to experiment. The lessons you'll learn along the way, the things you'll see, the obstacles you'll overcome, and the people you'll meet are more than enough reason to embark on this journey.

I like to end most of my projects with a call to action, and this one will take the form of a challenge. Find an ultramarathon within the next year. Sign up for it *today*. Start training *today*. To stay motivated, tell friends. Once you start training, join a local running group. If you need a wider social support network and have a high tolerance for dumbassery, feel free to look me up on Facebook (*www.facebook.com/robillardj*) and Twitter (*www.twitter.com/barefootjason*). I have a strong network of trail running and ultrarunning friends of all abilities and experience levels. They're a helpful bunch that can help you take the plunge into this great sport. A year from now when you're crossing the finish line, you will thank yourself for having the courage to take the plunge!

Good luck, friends!